menopause

menopause

the change for
the better

Written by expert
contributors and Henpicked

GREEN TREE
LONDON • OXFORD • NEW YORK • NEW DELHI • SYDNEY

GREEN TREE
Bloomsbury Publishing Plc
50 Bedford Square, London, WC1B 3DP, UK

BLOOMSBURY, GREEN TREE and the Green Tree logo are trademarks of
Bloomsbury Publishing Plc

First published in 2016 as Menopause: The Change for the Better - A Henpicked Easy
Guide to Menopause by Goldcrest Books Int. Ltd.
First published in Great Britain 2016
This edition published 2018

A catalogue record for this book is available from the British Library

Library of Congress Cataloguing-in-Publication data has been applied for

ISBN: TPB: 978-1-4729-4873-1; eBook: 978-1-4729-4874-8

2 4 6 8 10 9 7 5 3 1

Typeset in Adobe Garamond Pro by Deanta Global Publishing Services, Chennai, India
Printed and bound in Great Britain by CPI Group (UK) Ltd, Croydon, CR0 4YY

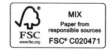

To find out more about our authors and books visit www.bloomsbury.com and
sign up for our newsletters

Contents

Foreword vii

Introduction 1

1 When will I start the menopause? 8

2 What is happening to my hormones? 21

3 What symptoms could I notice during menopause? 35

4 How will my periods be affected? 57

5 What happens to my bones and ligaments during menopause? 65

6 What is vaginal dryness and urinary incontinence? 78

7 What will happen to my sex drive? 94

8 Managing your menopause 108

9 What is 'premature' menopause? 140

10 Maintaining healthy relationships 157

11 Getting the best from your doctor's appointment 172

12 Menopause and work 180

13 Menopause: the time of your life 191

Glossary of Terms 193

Acknowledgements 197

Resources 206

Index 211

....

Life is for living...

Henpicked is a community website for women over 40. We often share menopause articles and some of the comments women write on our social media told us that there are lots of myths and misunderstandings about the menopause, with some women dreading it because of what they've heard or read, or having a bad time getting the help they want and need.

Before we wrote this guide, we carried out a survey and talked to groups of women. We found that there are lots of women who sail through it and lots who struggle. Along the way, we discovered the key questions women have about the menopause. So we decided to put this book together to provide easy-to-understand information. This is not designed to be a medical encyclopaedia or a tome of a book – just extra help, quick and easy to read at any time.

Many women tell us that they're happier after the menopause, so why not all of us? Why put up with symptoms if you do suffer with them, when you can do something about it? Or why wait until any symptoms get in the way of enjoying life?

Please don't be alarmed by headlines that can seem shocking when they hit out of the blue. The big headlines in 2002 about the safety of hormone replacement therapy (HRT) left many women not taking it because of the risks, based on research that was inaccurately reported to the media. Then again more recently, in 2016, another scary headline emerged without enough information for women to know if they are at risk or not. It's simply not on.

And being postmenopausal absolutely doesn't mean you're past it. Certainly not when you look at so many of the inspirational role models such as Helen Mirren and Judi Dench, who are successful, vibrant and glowing with life. And there are probably lots of women you know yourself. Many will tell you exactly how they feel about menopause if you ask.

We believe it's time to change the way we talk about the change. To dispel the myths, get to grips with the facts and talk about it more. We women are good at helping each other. Actually, that's what Henpicked's all about – sharing advice and tips and supporting each other. We believe we should talk about menopause more, with our partners, family, friends, managers and colleagues. Let's get menopause out in the open. So we talked to members of our community and experts and put this easy guide together. It won't take long to read but it does cover the key questions we get asked so you can understand it better. It tells you the important facts and if you read nothing else, you've made a very good start. And it shares women's personal experience.

There are resources in the back of the book about where you can find more information, and we'll keep sharing through Henpicked, too.

So get a drink of whatever you like and we hope you enjoy this book and join us in talking more about menopause.

The Henpicked team

Introduction

'Coming out of menopause is like a chrysalis becoming a butterfly, but this time with more experience.'
Anne Loadman

Menopause is a big thing. It's a transition in our lives, signalling the end of one era and the beginning of the next. One of the beauties of menopause is that it's your own, and your experience will be different to everyone else's. You may experience certain symptoms, issues and sometimes complications. Or you may not. For some women it takes over their lives, while others simply sail through it.

WHO IS THIS BOOK FOR?

We've noticed that there are countless books about puberty, pregnancy and childbirth, and about what to expect much later in life. But for some unfathomable reason, it isn't the same when it comes to menopause. Yes, there are some books and information, but we've found they often focus on the negatives or are too long or medical.

It's almost a taboo: women all over the world go through menopause, but it's not often something we discuss over a glass of wine. Yet it's a natural part of life for women. We all experience it at different times and in different ways. It's time to welcome in a new chapter of your life, with lots to look forward to. Your periods stop, but the world doesn't.

That's why we decided to write this easy guide. To share with you what you might expect, discuss the symptoms you could experience, and give you some food for thought. Our menopause experts, along with women from all walks of life, will be discussing their thoughts, fears and tips.

It's not about telling you what's right or wrong. What works for one woman may not work for the next, so by giving you as much independent, unbiased information as possible, we can help you to make informed decisions and do what's right for you during menopause and beyond.

WHY DO SOME WOMEN DREAD THE MENOPAUSE?

Many women approach the menopause with a sense of dread. As one woman put it, 'When I was growing up my mum had early menopause and all I recall are adjectives like "mad, crazy woman", and now I'm inherently afraid.'

But it's very important to have a sense of perspective. While one woman may sail through menopause with barely a symptom, another may feel it's taken over her life. We want to get real about it. To bring you the stories, positive and negative, and to help you take control and keep the balance in your life.

WHY DON'T WE TALK ABOUT MENOPAUSE OPENLY?

Modern society in the Western world is a difficult place for menopausal women. Why? Because we're constantly fed images of youth and beauty being the aspiration, our fertile years defining us as women. Female celebrities are frequently derided as they age, criticised for gaining or losing weight, for greying hair and for anything other than a perfectly wrinkle-free face. Is it surprising so many of them go under the knife? And then the media jumps on them for having surgery.

We asked our community why they thought people were still afraid to talk about menopause. While some women found that it had never been an issue, others felt that fear and embarrassment played a big part, along with persistent negative language surrounding the subject. Some felt that culturally we are ingrained into valuing youth and fertility, and menopause is seen as a loss of these and therefore not something to be celebrated. And in formal environments, such as at work, many women felt it was absolutely not a subject they could happily discuss with colleagues and managers.

We talk about 'going through' menopause as if it's some gruelling challenge, and we can only relax when we're at the end. It's also known as 'the change', a term often used in a derogatory sense.

So we've added our own ending to this phrase – let's make it **the change for the better**.

Which is why we love the quote we've opened with. Since when was change a bad thing? Why can't we look at menopause as a transformation, a new beginning, a metamorphosis? Interestingly, in Japanese culture this is exactly the case. Their word for this stage of a woman's life is 'konenki' – 'ko' means renewal or regeneration, 'nen' means years and 'ki' means energy. Renewal years and energy – a much more positive way of describing it.

And while we in the Western world are lamenting menopause, some of us feeling invisible or written off as old and past it, in some parts of the world women positively look forward to their postmenopausal years. In Mayan Indian tribes, for example, they can enjoy a new status in their communities, becoming the 'wise women' and leaders, revered for their life experiences.

YOUR QUESTIONS ANSWERED

In this book, we'll be exploring the physical and emotional aspects of all things menopause, answering some of the questions we've learned that women want the answers to. We've talked to women, lots of them! – and carried out focus groups, looked at feedback from articles posted on the Henpicked website and conducted our own survey. And these are the questions that kept cropping up.

We'll clarify the different stages of menopause, looking at the role that hormones play in our lives and how these change as we experience menopause. We'll examine the potential symptoms you might notice, and how to handle these, as well as giving you stories from women who are postmenopausal and loving it.

You'll find information about your options for support, from HRT through to alternative and natural methods. We've also included a chapter on how to get the best from your doctor and what to do if you feel you need more answers than your GP is giving you. Our chapter on menopause and work explains how you can cope if your symptoms are affecting you at work, and we also take a look at the effect it can have on your relationships with partners, family, colleagues and friends.

Finally, there are resources at the end of the book to point you to specific guidance for your own situation. As with anything health related, you need to take responsibility to figure out what works for you. This means arming yourself with as much information as possible about what you can do, what others can do to help you and where you can find support if and when you need it.

We're not pretending that menopause is something it isn't. But we are standing up and saying it's a natural process in a woman's life, like puberty, periods and pregnancy, and it's time for women to see it as a life phase, not as the end of their womanhood.

We hope you'll find this book informative, useful and above all, reassuring.

'In gambling they say that one hot flush is worth a million dollars. I say I'd rather have the million dollars please.'
Sue Hayes

OUR MENOPAUSE TEAM

This guide is written by Henpicked, an online community for women. It has been written with advice, information and input from experts in women's health and menopause.

We have a wealth of informative articles on the Henpicked website, and our aim is to give women a space to share their thoughts, ideas, advice and guidance on a wide range of topics. We've written this book as a result of women in our community telling us they'd like more accessible and understandable information about menopause. One of our members, Denise Hunt, told us she'd like 'a more practical book written by pragmatic women who have a sense of humour and are positive about what, actually, is a positive stage in a woman's life'.

In this guide, Henpicked is aiming to offer you an unbiased range of options and opinions. It's a personal choice and we urge you to explore in more detail anything in which you are interested. Expert opinion and advice may occasionally differ, and it's for you to decide which path is for you. There isn't a one-size-fits-all answer, and many women choose to combine a range of approaches. We don't endorse or recommend a particular approach, product or specialist, we simply describe it.

What we do want to do is offer every woman the chance to take control of her menopause.

We're not here to preach... it's over to you to read, absorb, research and decide.

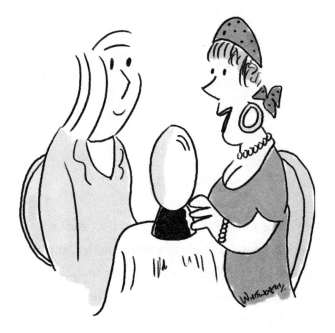

"YOU'RE ABOUT TO GO ON A
MYSTERIOUS JOURNEY."

When will I start the menopause?

'Perimenopause is not a short period of transition. And hormones do seriously affect your life.'
Lytisha Tunbridge

The word 'menopause' is rather misleading and a little misunderstood. While we talk about being menopausal and going through menopause, there are in fact different stages that make up the whole process, a series of gradual changes as your body adjusts to your shifting hormones.

Menopause is a biological stage in every woman's life that happens when you stop menstruating and reach the end of your natural reproductive life. It is when you have not had a period for 12 consecutive months (for women reaching menopause naturally).

The time leading up to the end of your periods is known as the perimenopause ('peri' meaning 'around'). The perimenopause is the time when you are still having periods but they may be changing in frequency or nature, and you may start to experience menopausal symptoms. This is when your body starts to prepare for menopause and changes start to happen.

You are in perimenopause right up until when you've not had a period for 12 consecutive months. Then the magical day happens – you know you have achieved menopause – the menopause is only one day in time. After that day, you are postmenopausal.

In this chapter, we will outline what types of changes you might notice and when. But you won't necessarily experience one stage, finish it, and move on to the next – they flow into each other as an organic process.

We think of menopause as being for women in their 40s and 50s, but some women will experience it much earlier, either through medical intervention or because of a natural early menopause. We'll also explore what impacts this can have and how to manage them. Menopause before the age of 40 is referred to as Premature Ovarian Insufficiency (POI). See our chapter **What is 'premature' menopause** for more on this.

WHEN DOES IT HAPPEN?

The average age for a woman in the UK to reach menopause is 51. For the majority of us, perimenopausal symptoms start at around the age of 45. For some women, this can begin as early as their 20s and for some as late as their late 40s or early 50s. It can start as late as a woman's early 60s, though this is very unusual.

It's a good idea to be aware of possible changes during this time. But you're very unlikely to be blasted with all the symptoms – indeed, you might put your symptoms down to your regular PMS (premenstrual syndrome), or just start to notice some changes in your monthly cycle.

WHEN DOES IT END?

You have reached menopause when you've gone 12 months with no periods. But this doesn't necessarily mean an end to all your symptoms – for example, you might still experience hot flushes for many years, even decades. Menopause symptoms usually last between four and eight years. There isn't really a defined start and end point.

WHAT COULD INFLUENCE THE AGE AT WHICH MENOPAUSE BEGINS?

There are certain factors that could influence the age at which you're likely to notice menopausal symptoms. These include:

The age your mother reached menopause

As menopause can be genetically linked, you're likely to follow a similar path. It's worth looking at the other women in your family too, such as your grandmother and aunts. If there's a strong pattern of similarities, then you're probably going to be around the same age.

If you smoke

You're more likely to reach menopause earlier than non-smokers.

Your ethnicity

Studies have shown this can sometimes have an effect. Chinese and Japanese women tend to reach their menopause a little later than European women, whereas Hispanic and African-American women experience their menopause a little earlier.

Ovarian surgery

Having your ovaries removed during an operation leads to an immediate menopause. If you have had your womb (uterus) removed – an operation called a hysterectomy – before your menopause, you may experience an early menopause, even if your ovaries are not removed. Although your ovaries will still make some oestrogen after a hysterectomy, it is common that your level of oestrogen will fall at an earlier age than average. As you do not have periods after a hysterectomy, it may not be clear when you are menopausal. However, you are likely to develop some typical symptoms when your level of oestrogen falls. See chapter two for more on oestrogen.

Symptoms can actually be more severe than if you had a natural menopause, as your oestrogen levels drop abruptly.

Chemotherapy

Some types of chemotherapy and radiotherapy can cause an early menopause. Your cycles may return to normal when you've finished treatment, but you're still likely to reach menopause a few years earlier than you would have otherwise.

You might be surprised to learn what *doesn't* have any influence on your menopause. The age at which you have your first period, for example, has no bearing. Some women think that they have a certain number of cycles, but this isn't the case. Similarly, if you've been pregnant or have breastfed, this won't have any effect. And using hormonal birth control has also not been shown to have any impact on when you begin to enter perimenopause.

WHAT SYMPTOMS MIGHT INDICATE PERIMENOPAUSE?

It's worth knowing what's on the list, because if you notice a few of these symptoms you'll have an idea of what's happening. And actually, these are both perimenopausal and menopausal symptoms.

Changes in cycle length

Although you may notice that your periods become less frequent and lighter, some women find that their periods become closer together and sometimes heavier as they approach the menopause.

Sudden onset or worsening symptoms of PMS

Some women find a worsening of their PMS symptoms, such as bloating, irritability, food cravings, mood swings and lethargy. These symptoms are usually due to the fluctuating levels of hormones that occur in your body.

Hot flushes

These are the most common symptom of the menopause and occur in around three out of four women. They usually come on very suddenly and spread through your body, chest, neck and face. They vary in length from a few minutes to much longer. They can be associated with symptoms such as sweating, dizziness, light-headedness and even heart palpitations. They can occur many times throughout the day and can continue for many years – some women even experience hot flushes later in life, in their 70s and 80s. They usually occur spontaneously but can come on after eating certain types of food or drinking alcohol, especially wine.

Night sweats

These can also be very common and very troublesome. Many women find they wake up several times each night and are drenched in sweat, needing to change their bedclothes and bed linen. This can obviously be very disruptive to their partner, too.

Changes in sex drive

Reduced or absent libido (sex drive) occurs when your hormone levels fall. This can also be related to low testosterone levels in your body.

Sleep disturbance

This can be related to disrupted sleep from night sweats but many women also find that they have a more unsettled and less fulfilled night's sleep when they are perimenopausal. Even if your sleep is not affected, you may find that you are more tired than normal during the day.

Weight gain

You might notice some extra weight, in particular around your middle.

Breast pain

As with your period or pregnancy, changes in your hormones during perimenopause can cause sore or swollen breasts.

Mood changes

Not all women experience mood swings but for some women they can be very disruptive. They can be more common if you have had PMS in the past.

Memory problems

It can be common to forget words, appointments and birthdays and even to do odd things (for example, put your car keys in the fridge!). Many women find that their brain does not feel as engaged as it used to and this can really affect their ability to work and function.

Vaginal dryness, itching or soreness

The lack of oestrogen in your body tends to cause the tissues around your vagina to become thinner, drier and inflamed. These changes can take months or even years to develop and vary between women. Your vagina may shrink a little and expand less easily during sex, making sexual intercourse more painful or uncomfortable.

Your vulva may become thin, dry and itchy. You may notice that your vulva or vagina has become red and sore. You may also find you have episodes of thrush more frequently. Many women have symptoms of vaginal pain and discomfort throughout the day, so it is often not just a problem to those women who are sexually active.

As the skin around your vagina becomes more sensitive, it is more likely to itch. This can make you prone to scratching, which then makes your skin more likely to itch, and so on.

Hair and skin changes

Although your skin can change as you become older anyway, the changes in your hormone levels can lead to additional changes to your skin. Oestrogen is important for building collagen, the protein that supports the structure of your skin. Lower levels of oestrogen can lead to skin changes such as reduced elasticity, dryness, fine wrinkling and your skin becoming thinner. Some women find their skin becomes itchier. Acne and increased facial hair growth can occur in some women during the menopause too, again due to an imbalance of hormones.

Oestrogen is very important for your hair growth so you may notice that your hair becomes thinner and less glossy.

Worsening migraines

If you have had migraines in the past, you may find that they become more severe or closer together. This can be a sign that your hormone levels are changing.

Poor concentration

It is common to find that you do not concentrate as well as you used to. Many women find that it is harder to multitask and this can be very frustrating.

Urinary symptoms

The low levels of oestrogen in your body can lead to thinning and weakening of the tissues around the neck of your bladder, or around the opening for urine to pass (your urethra). For example, urinary symptoms that may occur include an urgency to get to the toilet and recurring urinary tract infections (UTIs) or cystitis.

Depression, anxiety, panic attacks and irritability

Emotional symptoms during the perimenopause and menopause can really vary between women. Some women find that symptoms of depression, anxiety, panic attacks, anger and irritation worsen so much that they really interfere with the quality of their life. These symptoms can affect your emotional well-being and add to the stress of life in general.

Joint and muscle pain

Lower oestrogen levels can sometimes lead to joint and muscle pain, as oestrogen can have an anti-inflammatory effect and also helps to make cartilage.

Obviously, not everything that affects us between the ages of 45 and 65 is menopausal in origin.

If a symptom worries you then listen to your intuition and see a medical professional.

IS THERE ANY WAY TO CONFIRM WHETHER I'M GOING THROUGH THE MENOPAUSE?

If you're over 45 and have irregular periods with symptoms of the menopause then you don't need to have any tests, including hormone blood tests, to diagnose menopause. The diagnosis is made by your symptoms alone. If you are taking contraception or have a Mirena coil, which is a type of coil containing progestogen, it may be difficult to know what your periods are like.

If you're under 45 and experiencing symptoms of the menopause, your doctor may decide that you need to have tests. The most common is a blood test measuring the level of follicle stimulating hormone (FSH). This is the hormone that regulates the amount of oestrogen in your body. If you have low levels of oestrogen, your FSH level is usually raised – if this is the case, it is very likely that you are menopausal. This blood test is often repeated four to six weeks later. However, as hormone levels can fluctuate, some women are menopausal despite a normal FSH level.

For some women, being on the pill or having hormonal implants has already stopped their periods, so it's not always clear if they've gone into menopause or not. If you feel it's important to know, from a contraceptive point of view, speak to your GP. If you are menopausal, you will still need to use contraception for two years after your last period if you're under 50 and one year if you're over 50. It can be helpful to make a note of the date of your last period.

If you're under 45 years of age, you should certainly not be told you are or are not menopausal on the strength of one blood test.

There is no test available to determine when your menopause is actually going to happen, so it's not always easy to diagnose where you are on your menopause journey. Sorry! What is worth doing is reading what's in this book, understanding how you feel and tracking your periods.

I'VE MISSED A PERIOD. AM I IN MENOPAUSE?

Your periods are likely to become irregular as you enter the perimenopausal phase. You might notice your cycle becomes less predictable, your flow changes and yes, you might start missing some periods.

Stress is a common trigger for missed periods – at any age – as is weight loss or gain. You can still become pregnant, even with erratic periods, so remember to use contraception.

POSTMENOPAUSE

You are postmenopausal the day after you reach menopause. However, many women continue to experience menopausal symptoms such as hot flushes, night sweats and vaginal dryness for many years or even decades.

WOMEN'S STORIES...

'I always used to look upon the menopause as a far-off thing that happens when a woman gets old. But, during my homeopathic training, I realised there's a lot more to menopause than meets the eye. I was shocked to discover how massive the changes can be – I'd never even considered there would be emotional issues alongside the more obvious physical changes.

Emotions are often linked to other problems surrounding health and well-being, so if you're able to find ways to stop yourself hanging on to grudges, regrets, anger and other emotional baggage earlier in life, you should have an easier ride when your hormones start to adjust.

I developed heavy periods and fibroids in my mid-40s. I believe in the benefits of homeopathy and my homeopath prescribed remedies that triggered my body to heal and I didn't need the threatened surgery. It also eliminated the extreme period pain I had suffered all my adult years (and my mother before me). If only I had known that was possible when I was younger!

Then some unfinished business crawled out of the woodwork. Raw, empty feelings of loss and bereavement appeared as my periods reduced in frequency.

My childbearing years were coming to an end and something that had always been a possibility for me, a child of my own, was no more. That instinct, the desire I'd thought had been laid to rest, ignited itself again. I knew it was crazy and impossible for so many reasons but my heart and body yearned for quite a while. Only when the final periods faded into distant memory did I truly find peace again.

My fulfilling career suddenly stopped firing me up. Slowly a realisation that there was another way came to me. It was time to put myself, my needs and dreams first in my life.

My career had for so long been my stability, the thing that I escaped to during hard times, the job title was who I was. Changing that was no small step.

Sometimes life gives us a big push or, if we are lucky, it dangles an opportunity in a glaringly obvious way. In my case, this was voluntary redundancy. My heart wanted me to be at home walking my dogs and feeling in balance. Part of me was terrified but I took the redundancy and soon my future was a blank canvas and it felt good.

A few months on, working part time, I took a life-changing trip to Peru and was drawn to train in the Andean Shamanic Energy Medicine. Then I also trained as a homeopath. I was being taken somewhere and fast! But where?

Suddenly I moved into a new phase. Now there was time to apply and deepen what I had learned for the benefit of others.

Finding a new purpose in life and doing what fires and delights us is so important. Only then can we contribute to the lives of those around us. For me, as for many others, it is a truly creative passion and a deep-seated urge to do "what I do".

Earlier in life we are often told that is selfish yet with that wisdom age brings the realisation that it is essential, like breathing, for us to stay truly alive and vibrant.'

Carol Fieldhouse

2

....

What is happening to my hormones?

'I want to let women know that it doesn't have to be awful.'
Sally Mayes

Many people talk about feeling hormonal during menopause, saying things like 'my hormones are all over the place' or 'it must be my hormones' as a catch-all phrase to explain why they're feeling the way they are. But although your hormones will change, that doesn't mean that you have to just put up or shut up. Your body is going through an amazing transformation. If puberty is a time for hormones to come alive, menopause certainly isn't a time for them to die. It's a time for them to evolve.

There's a symphony of hormones at play throughout your life. When your hormones are balanced, you generally feel good. But when the balance of your hormones changes – as it will during perimenopause – that's when you often experience problems.

Below, we explain some of the symptoms you might notice with both excessive and declining hormone levels, and you may find that some of these symptoms overlap. The key is to find your own way to restore some balance to your hormones. Hormonal balance and preservation of your remaining hormones is important to help you through your perimenopausal years and beyond.

While you can't avoid the natural transition into menopause, there are certainly plenty of things you can do to help yourself as your hormones begin their sometimes wayward journey of change. And as with most things, forewarned is forearmed. In the same way that it's a good idea to have an understanding of your menstrual cycle, knowing what's happening to your body during menopause can help you make the right decisions for you to restore some balance.

This chapter looks at the different hormones at play during menopause, what their functions are, and what changes you might experience as a result.

OESTROGEN

Oestrogen – or estrogen, the US spelling – is the hormone most commonly associated with women. And if you've spotted signs of the perimenopause or you're further along your menopausal journey, you'll probably have discovered that the levels of this powerful hormone play a vital role in how you look and feel.

Perhaps you've come across claims that your ovaries just 'fail' one day and your oestrogen levels take a nosedive towards oblivion and disappear once your body approaches the menopause. But it's all rather more complex than that.

What does oestrogen do?

This hormone is responsible for lots of processes in your body. It:

- Triggers the 'ripening' and release of an egg every month, ready for fertilisation.
- Stops the release of follicle stimulating hormones (FSH) so that only one egg is released.
- Nourishes the tissues of the body with blood and keeps them youthful and elastic, including the tissue of your skin and your vagina.
- Regulates new bone turnover and cholesterol levels.
- Keeps your organs such as your brain, liver and heart healthy.
- Maintains your brainpower by affecting your levels of acetylcholine, a neurotransmitter associated with neuron growth and with memory and learning. Throughout your reproductive years, it's mostly produced in your ovaries, then after the menopause, when ovulation no longer occurs, your fatty tissue, breast tissue, liver and adrenals take over the role, producing lower levels of this hormone.

Did you know there are three main types of oestrogen?

The three main types of oestrogen each work differently in the body. If you're more familiar with the US spellings, we've added these here too, for clarity – the spellings are different but the definitions are exactly the same.

1. Oestradiol/estradiol

This is the strongest and most active form of oestrogen. It is produced in your ovaries and is responsible for changes during puberty and your menstrual cycle. When we discuss perimenopausal oestrogen levels, we are usually referring to this one.

2. Oestrone/estrone

At the time of the menopause itself, our bodies begin to produce oestrone – another form of oestrogen, which our bodies convert to oestradiol. This hormone is produced in your ovaries while they are still operational, then switch to your fatty tissue, liver and adrenals. Unlike oestradiol, oestrone doesn't fluctuate on a monthly basis and is significantly weaker.

3. Oestriol/estriol

This is a by-product of oestradiol and oestrone and it is mainly made in your liver. It is also produced by the placenta during pregnancy. It is the weakest form of oestrogen.

What happens to our oestrogen levels during the menopause?

The hormones oestrogen and progesterone work together in your body to regulate your menstrual cycle. During your perimenopause, the levels of these hormones fluctuate greatly and it is often the imbalance of these hormones that leads to menopausal symptoms occurring.

PROGESTERONE

It's easy to fall into the trap of thinking menopause is about oestrogen and ovaries and nothing else, but there are other powerful hormones at play during this time, too. One of the primary hormones is progesterone, which plays an important role in the health of your reproductive system and how balanced your hormones are as a whole. It also helps keep your oestrogen levels in check.

What does progesterone do?

Progesterone plays a number of important roles. It:

- Boosts natural feelings of calmness.
- Helps you to enjoy relaxing, rejuvenating sleep.
- Increases your pain threshold.
- Helps normalise blood sugar levels.
- Can improve your mood.
- Plays a central role in achieving and maintaining pregnancy.

Progesterone is produced in your ovaries after you ovulate, in the placenta during pregnancy and in smaller amounts in the adrenal glands.

What happens to our progesterone levels during menopause?

Progesterone plays an opposing role to oestrogen, helping it to achieve balance and keeping tissue growth in check. Throughout the course of your menstrual cycle, these hormones are in perfect balance, first oestrogen rising in the weeks leading up to ovulation, then progesterone taking over until your period arrives. But during the perimenopause, this doesn't happen. The relative balance of progesterone and oestrogen changes, making your cycle less predictable.

TESTOSTERONE

Generally associated with men, testosterone is actually a vital hormone for women, too – in fact, women produce three times as much testosterone as oestrogen. The difference is that females produce a nifty enzyme called aromatase, which converts the majority of this testosterone into oestrogen. It's primarily made in your ovaries, adrenal glands and body fat.

What does testosterone do?

Testosterone plays a vital role in helping us look and feel our best. It:

- Keeps you motivated and optimistic.
- Makes you feel brighter and more assertive.
- Helps you enjoy a satisfying sex life.
- Supports and increases bone density.
- Turns fat into muscle.
- Helps to improve cognitive function.
- Helps to keep your liver and heart healthy.

What happens to testosterone during the menopause?

As you enter your menopausal years, your natural levels of testosterone reduce, especially in women who have had their ovaries removed.

For many women, this lowering of testosterone, along with low oestrogen levels, can bring with it the following symptoms: low moods, depression, lack of motivation, lower sex drive, fatigue, reduced muscle tone, decrease in bone density (which can lead to osteoporosis) and a reduction in muscle tone in your bladder and pelvis, which can lead to urinary incontinence and a weakening of genital tissues.

GETTING THE RIGHT BALANCE

If your fluctuating hormones are getting you down, you'll be pleased to know there are steps you can take to feel more balanced. There's no 'right' way of doing it, you need to find what works best for you. Whether it's speaking to a doctor or a menopause expert, making adjustments to your lifestyle, taking HRT or a combination of medical and natural solutions, you don't need to suffer with the problems that wayward hormones can bring.

Life's for living, so please don't feel you just have to put up with symptoms. There are solutions!

THE NATURAL APPROACH

There's plenty you can do to help yourself. Depending on your lifestyle, it might just mean a few tweaks here or there, or you may need to make some bigger changes. If you feel daunted, just try to introduce one thing at a time. You'll soon notice a difference in the way you feel.

Tackle your stress levels

When you're stressed, your cortisol (stress hormone) levels shoot up, which in turn can interfere with the balance of oestrogen and progesterone in your body.

The best way to tackle this is to choose your favourite relaxation technique and indulge, whether that means taking long hot baths with a great book, yoga, meditation, chatting with friends or enjoying your favourite hobby.

Eat cholesterol and fats

Although we've been conditioned to avoid cholesterol in our diets, it's actually essential for producing testosterone and making new cell membranes. This isn't a green light to eat cakes though (sorry!), as we're talking about good fats here. You'll find these in foods like avocado, oily fish and eggs.

Enjoy phytoestrogens

Phytoestrogens became of interest to scientists because they realised that women in certain traditional cultures like that of Japan, who eat a diet rich in these plant foods have fewer menopausal symptoms than Western women.*

*Nagata, C. *et al*, 2001, 'Soy product intake and hot flushes in Japanese women: results from a community based prospective study', Am. J. Epidem., 153, 790-793.

These are plant-based foods that exert a naturally oestrogenic effect upon your body. Great sources include oats, barley, beans, lentils, yams, rice, alfalfa and mung beans.

Take some exercise
This is really essential for keeping your hormones balanced. If you've never exercised before, or not in a while, then take it slowly at first rather than rushing in head first. Try to find something you enjoy, as you're more likely to stick with it. Aim for about 30 minutes three times a week.

Spend time outdoors
Whether it's sunny or dull, being outside and getting some light can really help to restore your balance. It's not just about going for a 'nice walk' or 'getting a bit of fresh air'. Your circadian rhythms help to regulate core body temperature, hormonal processes, cell regeneration and much more. Without light, our rhythm goes out of whack, we feel down and dull, and our metabolic, hormonal, sleeping and eating patterns and central nervous system can all change and alter glucose production. In essence, light fuels our body, helping it to function well, and if we don't get enough we feel sad and tired. It will also boost your levels of vitamin D, essential for helping our bodies to absorb calcium – which in turn can help to reduce the risk of osteoporosis. It is really difficult for most women to get enough vitamin D from sunlight alone all year round. The current recommendation for everyone over the age of one is to take 10mcg of vitamin D every day.

Balance your blood sugar levels

High blood sugar triggers a release of insulin, which stresses your entire endocrine system – a collection of glands that produce hormones that regulate metabolism, growth and development, tissue function, sexual function, reproduction, sleep and mood – and can inhibit the production of oestrogen. Try to cut out processed sugars and opt for healthier alternatives. It will really help.

Support your liver

Your liver metabolises waste oestrogen and ensures its production after the menopause, so it's clearly vital for hormonal health. To keep it working optimally, ditch processed foods, especially those that are high in processed fat, and reduce your alcohol intake.

THE MEDICAL APPROACH

We've outlined some of the natural ideas for balancing your hormones, and we'll talk more about diet and exercise in our **Managing your menopause** chapter.

There are also medical treatments you can try, either in conjunction with natural methods or in isolation. Again, we'll explore these in greater detail in **Managing your menopause**.

HORMONE REPLACEMENT THERAPY (HRT)

HRT is available as tablets, skin patches or gel. There are different types and strengths of treatment, but all will contain oestrogen. HRT can help to restore your hormonal balance and relieve some of the unpleasant symptoms you may be experiencing. As well as reducing your hot flushes and controlling your mood swings, it can also help to reduce your risk of heart attack and stroke, strengthen your bones and improve the look of your hair and skin.

Some women take HRT for a short period of time to help them get through their menopausal symptoms. Other women feel so great on it, and want to maximise the cardiovascular benefit and reduce their osteoporosis risk, that they continue to take HRT for a longer time.

The length of time to take HRT is an individual decision that should be made after discussion with your GP or menopause expert.

THE MIRENA COIL

This is an intrauterine system that acts as a contraceptive, releasing progesterone into the uterus. If you're suffering from heavy or prolonged bleeding, this is a good option to help reduce or even eradicate your periods. You can use a coil as a contraceptive or in conjunction with HRT.

If you're worried or would like advice about any of your symptoms, please speak to your GP or a menopause expert.

'Learn more about sex. It could be the best time and gift of your life.'
Mayarita

WOMEN'S STORIES...

"'I'm getting old," "I'm drying up" and "I'm giving up." These are comments I regularly hear from women who are approaching menopause.

Of course, you may be one of those women who are happy with yourself and have positive thoughts and feelings about getting older.

Whichever camp you fall in, you can learn to change your perspective, or take your positivity to the next level and even feel excited about this new chapter in your life.

In the ancient tripartite divisions, it is said that there are three stages of life for women: Maiden, Mother and Crone. Each stage represents a gateway in life.

Menopause is in the Crone (or Wise Woman) stage, when a woman's 'wise blood' remains inside her to give her wisdom.

In Neolithic times, Crone women were the matriarchs. Their connection to the Earth, along with their wisdom gained through their lineage and ancestors, made them valued and honoured by their community. Unfortunately, this isn't always the case in society nowadays, as more value seems to be placed on looks and material possessions.

We are living in an extremely powerful time in history where we can make the changes necessary to enhance not only our lives but we can give back to life all that we have learned.

We can use our voice for the highest good by speaking our truth and leading by example. As Wise Women, we can be a light for our daughters and sons by teaching them what we have learned and guiding them to trust their own instincts. And we can fully step into our potency knowing that we have lived a rich and rewarding life.

The hormonal shifts that occur at the time of menopause can bring about powerful changes in your life. Some women think of it as a message from their bodies – telling them they are coming to the end of their caretaking duties. The physical symptoms remind us to consider our own needs too.

I know from experience that this is extremely challenging for many women as we are literally wired up to nurture and look after others.

There may also be a period of grieving as you have the choice to let go of certain aspects from your past. All the regrets and things you wished you had said and done.

For those of us that have children, we may see them grow up and leave the nest.

But most of all, it is also the most wonderful opportunity to start a new chapter.

Many women do find it hard to become so self-aware suddenly but there's so much we can do to identify which areas of your health and life you can improve as you approach menopause. It's not all doom and gloom, there's lots to look forward to and lots you can do.

As we are becoming healthier and living longer, we can truly embrace our lives and look forward to a future filled with zest, youthfulness and vitality.'

Kim Rossi

....

3

What symptoms could I notice during menopause?

'It was liberating for me, but for friends it's been really hard – every woman experiences the menopause differently.'
Deborah Granville

Around eight out of ten women experience some menopausal symptoms, and around 25 per cent of women have very severe symptoms. More than half of women have menopausal symptoms for more than seven years. In this chapter, we'll explore some of the changes you might start to notice, and what you can do to ease them.

But before we do that, there are two important things to say:
If you haven't gone through menopause yet, or are perimenopausal, it's important to realise that not every woman will notice every symptom we describe here. Menopause is a

personal thing and your body won't respond in the same way as another woman's. So please, please, please don't feel alarmed and start thinking the worst.

If you are suffering or something is worrying you or causing difficulty, you should make an appointment to see your doctor or menopause expert. Not everything you experience while you're going through menopause can be put down as a 'symptom of ageing'.

WHAT ARE HOT FLUSHES AND HOW CAN I PREVENT THEM?

Hot flushes – or flashes – are one of the 'classic' symptoms that many people associate with menopause. And you'll know when one arrives, as you'll feel overcome with heat, your make-up can start sliding off and your clothes can stick to your skin. Lovely!

During menopause, some women feel as if their thermostats have gone haywire. This is caused by your fluctuating hormone levels. You become suffused with heat and sweat, and flush in order to cool down. Sometimes this happens too quickly and you start to shiver and shake. For some women, this is one of the defining symptoms of menopause. Others wonder what all the fuss is about.

Hot flushes tend to last for about four minutes on average. You could get them as often as every hour to just a few times a week. You'll usually notice them on your head, face, neck and chest, and they can often disrupt your sleep patterns.

So what can you do about them?

THE MEDICAL APPROACH

As hot flushes are caused by your hormone levels, eating spicy foods won't cause (or indeed relieve) hot flushes. But some women do find these foods, or drinking alcohol, especially wine, can make their flushes worse. HRT is the most effective treatment available to improve your hot flushes and, at the right doses, stops them in over 95 per cent of women. For some women, other drugs such as antidepressants can improve hot flushes.

For more on HRT, see our chapter on **Managing your menopause.**

THE NATURAL APPROACH

If you've decided not to take HRT, you may choose to try to tackle your hot flushes the natural way. Making some lifestyle adjustments can help to combat them. Reducing stress is a big one. While this isn't always easy as many of us have busy lives, it really is worth trying. Why? Because when you're stressed you release cortisol, which can upset your hormonal balance and exacerbate any symptoms you're already having.

Self-hypnosis can help, using positive visualisation and relaxation techniques. You might also find yoga or meditation helps you to switch off and wind down for a while. Learning breathing techniques is a good idea – in yoga, belly breathing is a technique for relaxation.

Exercise is good for you and it's easier to do something that you enjoy because you're more likely to keep it up. Try to aim for three 30-minute sessions a week.

But some forms of exercise are better than others, particularly if you're finding your existing regime is no longer working and you're piling the pounds on around your middle. Our personal training experts agree that high intensity interval training (HIIT) is particularly good for menopausal women and reducing abdominal fat. This consists of exercising at an intensity that keeps your heart rate high and taking short breaks between each workout interval so your heart rate doesn't drop too much. It gets your heart racing and makes you feel sweaty (yes, there's the irony!) but long term it can help with balancing your hormones. This type of exercise is different to traditional cardio – there are some schools of thought that these are not appropriate for menopausal women because traditional cardio is thought to increase cortisol levels for longer periods than HIIT and raised cortisol is linked to weight gain.

However, you'll find information about different types of exercise in our **What happens to my bones and ligaments during menopause?** and **Managing your menopause** chapters.

Cleaning up your diet can also help. This isn't about jumping on a faddy diet bandwagon, more about introducing real (rather than processed) foods into your diet, and thinking about how different foods make you feel after you've eaten them. Keep your blood sugar balanced with plenty of protein and eat regular meals.

While some women don't mind the occasional sweaty spell, for others it can really inhibit their lives, making them embarrassed in social or professional situations.

Whether you prefer a natural or medical approach, or a combination of the two, you can start to tackle the hot flushes and make them a manageable part of your menopause.

WHY DO I FEEL SO EMOTIONAL?

While we tend to focus on the physical side of menopause, the emotional side is often just as turbulent.

Do you find yourself crying helplessly one minute and shouting furiously the next? While some are less affected than others, it's undeniably the case that your changing hormones can cause some difficult mood swings.

You might find yourself erupting over the slightest thing, becoming more prone to road rage, arguing more with your partner or children. And it's tough because you don't want to feel like this and you know your hormones are to blame. But you don't want to risk alienating your friends and loved ones, just at the time you really need their support.

WHAT CAUSES THE MOOD SWINGS?

If you've ever suffered from PMS, you'll understand the intensity of the emotions you can experience as a result of changing hormone levels.

It's a similar story when it comes to the menopause. When you enter the perimenopausal years, your ovaries function less efficiently than before, leading to imbalances in many of your hormones, including oestrogen, progesterone and testosterone. This affects your brain chemistry and as a result you might feel more irritable, angry, depressed and emotional than before. This helps to explain why you can feel fine one minute then ready to cry (or scream) the next.

IS IT NORMAL THAT I WANT TO SPEND MORE TIME ALONE?

Historically, menopause has been associated with loss and decline, leading to much of the negativity, fear and apprehension that still surrounds it. Today there are more postmenopausal women on the planet than there have ever been and the average life expectancy for a woman is now into her 80s. This has resulted in women starting to explore, speak and write about the profound shift that can occur at this point in their lives, resulting in a powerful transformation to the next stage of life rather than an ending.

Your emotions are always encouraging you to get your needs met. During perimenopause, many women report a strong yearning to retreat to a place of sanctuary, away from the world and their everyday responsibilities. To be free of the distractions that come with caring for others to focus upon their own needs and simply to reflect on the past, consider the future, and just be.

So it's quite common to feel the deep desire to retreat from everyday life and spend some time in solitude with no one to please and no interruptions to your peace and quiet. Menopause should be a time of self-care, but in today's fast-paced environment that can prove to be difficult, sometimes impossible, so we need to make time to care for ourselves.

The first step is simply acknowledging this inner voice, accepting that at this time in your life you are being urged to make some time for reflection. This can result in deep feelings of frustration and resentment when other responsibilities and perhaps lack of time or resources make this complete retreat impossible. The reality in today's society is that for most women this prolonged retreat is simply out of reach from our busy lives. So if several weeks or months in your ideal location with no distractions is simply not a possibility for you, rest assured that there are many things you can do to promote self-care and compassion at this time of transition.

THE NATURAL APPROACH

If you have been suffering with mood swings, the first thing to do is stop feeling ashamed of yourself and thinking that you're a 'bad person'. At the same time, take your head out of the sand, because just hoping things will resolve themselves is unlikely to help.

The solution comes down to you. Only you have the power to come to terms with your emotions; only you can overcome your anger.

The menopause can lead you to question your identity. It's a time of reassessment that can make you consider, reflect and review almost every aspect of your life. The way you perceive yourself begins to shift, but you're often not quite sure exactly what this means.

Are you no longer that young, energetic and sexy person? Are you somehow less feminine than before? Will your partner see you differently? What if you haven't completed your family yet? What will your friends think? Are you getting old? It's vital to work through all of these thoughts if you're ever to find inner peace. This takes time and patience.

The menopause also brings to light any pre-existing emotional or psychological issues that you haven't yet dealt with. Perhaps it's time to admit that your relationship isn't quite going the way you hoped, or that you feel lonely, or you hate your job. Times of crisis like these bring out the vulnerability in all of us, the emotional scars and the barriers that prevent us living life to our full potential.

Teamed with the biological chaos, it can often be a potent recipe for disaster – and at the same time, the perfect opportunity to heal.

LETTING GO OF THE RAGE

The first, and most important, step to take when dealing with your anger is to admit that you are suffering from it – otherwise, it will likely return in the future in bigger and scarier doses.

You will then be able to benefit from a wide range of psychological tools to help you tackle your anger, relieve any underlying stress, boost your self-esteem, lift your mood and help to clarify your thoughts.

These include things like:

- Positive visualisation
- Mindfulness meditation
- Neuro-Linguistic Programming (NLP) tools
- Deep-breathing exercises

Don't think you are alone if you are finding the menopause challenging to deal with. There are many women who are going through exactly the same thing as you and can offer the kind of support you need.

FINDING TIME FOR SELF-CARE AND REFLECTION

We all know how difficult it can be to find time for ourselves, and we've mentioned how hard it can be to physically take time out for long periods. But there are still ways to make things a little easier on yourself.

Listen to your inner voice

Your emotions are your inner guidance system, and understanding how your thoughts and emotions affect you and knowing how to change them in a positive way is empowering.

Breathe deeply

Breathing properly can make all the difference to the way you feel. It may sound strange – we breathe all the time, after all – but there are different techniques you can use to help you fully relax. This means breathing completely in and completely out each time – often we don't fully expel all the air from one breath before we take another, which can lead to a stressed-out, anxious feeling.

Belly breathing is great for relaxation. You might need to practise at first to help you get used to the technique. Try lying down on the floor and placing your hands on your belly. Inhale deeply, noticing your belly expand first. Then exhale for a longer count – so if you inhale for three seconds exhale for six to ten seconds – tightening your core and contracting your abdominal muscles. This will push your diaphragm back up.

With a little practice, you'll soon get used to this way of breathing and find it easier to relax.

Make time whenever you can

It might be a walk in the park, a cup of tea in the garden or time spent with a good book, but whatever you choose to do, make sure everybody around you knows that this is your time. Many women find it a challenge to take time out for themselves, particularly if they have lived a life of caring for others, but it really is vital to have some me time, however brief.

Become your own best friend

We can be very hard on ourselves – we berate ourselves for our mistakes, chastise ourselves for our failures and often speak to ourselves in very negative ways. Ask yourself, would I speak to my best friend in the same way? Of course you wouldn't, you would be kind and supportive and encouraging. The next time you find yourself saying anything to yourself that you wouldn't say to your best friend, stop and practise being a little kinder to yourself. The more we interrupt these negative thought patterns and challenge them with more positive thoughts, the less likely they are to occur automatically.

Take a yoga class

If you've never practised yoga before, now is the ideal time to start, as a gentle supportive restorative class can relieve joint pain and improve flexibility. The powerful breathing practices can be helpful in allowing you to control hot flushes and spend time more mindfully.

Seek support

There are times in our lives when we all need a little extra support. Showing your vulnerability is not a sign of weakness – it takes great courage to admit that we need help. Seek support from your friends and family, or speak to a professional therapist. Increasingly, women are gathering together to support each other and share their experiences and there is great therapeutic benefit in simply being heard.

Communicate

Many women speak about how unprepared they felt for menopause so it follows that partners and families are equally unprepared for the changes that may happen. It is important to keep the lines of communication open and to let loved ones know that we don't need them to fix us but just to be there for us, to listen, care and support.

Menopause Cafes are springing up around the country too. Their purpose is to give people the chance to talk to others in a social environment, raising awareness of menopause and understanding about the impact it can have. Check to see if there's one in your area or set one up yourself.

Keep a journal

Menopause can be a time of great transformation, of coming home to yourself. Hormonal changes can bring about a metamorphosis, and you may notice that you begin to focus on what is really important to you and strip away what no longer serves you. Starting a journal is a good way to record your thoughts as you begin to consider the future you really want at this next stage of your life.

It's always a good idea to consult a trained professional to help you find the best ways to tackle your emotional issues. See the **Resources** section at the end of this book.

THE MEDICAL APPROACH

If you feel that your mood swings aren't going away or that they are something more, then please go and see your GP or menopause expert. It's common for menopausal women to feel as if they're 'going mad'. Don't let yourself get to the point where you feel desperate – seek a medical opinion as soon as you start to feel something is amiss.

Menopause symptoms should never be shrugged off as something to simply bear. If your symptoms are affecting your life and your well-being and you feel you are losing control, it can start to seep into every area of your life and this is when relationships, family life and your work life can start to suffer.

Your GP may suggest cognitive behavioural therapy (CBT), a type of talking and behaviour modification therapy. CBT helps you to transform negative thought patterns and cycles, breaking your problems down into smaller, easier-to-manage parts. It is not a regressive therapy, in that it deals purely with the issues you're having now, rather than looking back at your past.

HRT can often really help with the mood changes that occur with the menopause. This is because it restores your levels of hormones and also keeps them at a constant level.

Your GP may also prescribe antidepressants if they feel you are suffering from clinical depression. In some cases, low doses can help to relieve other menopausal symptoms too, such as hot flushes, and can be especially helpful for women who cannot take HRT. However, the evidence for their effectiveness is poor and they often only work in the short term. As with all treatments, you'll need to talk it through thoroughly with your GP and make an informed decision about whether antidepressants are right for you. However, antidepressants should not be given instead of HRT.

HELP! WHY CAN'T I SEEM TO SHIFT THE FAT AROUND MY MIDDLE?

As we get older, it's perfectly normal to get a little wider around the middle. And the belly bulge can be something you're dreading as you approach menopause, especially if it's something you noticed with your own mother and even grandmother.

If you've noticed some extra pounds, you might have started to cut back on calories to shift the weight, or invested in some body-shaping underwear. Perhaps you've found yourself sucking your tummy in when you're getting undressed in front of your partner... sound familiar?

But once again, it's not just a case of hey-ho, I'm getting older so I'll never have a waistline again. Your metabolism hasn't come to a screeching halt overnight, nor are your genes responsible for your changing shape.

What causes the fat around the middle?

Firstly, your body is working extra hard to achieve hormonal balance as your oestrogen and progesterone levels are tapering off. And your changing hormones can have an effect on your weight and where your body stores fat. The drop in oestrogen tells your body to store excess pounds on your tummy instead of your bottom and thighs.

Secondly, these hormonal changes, and the way they make you feel – tense or anxious – send your stress hormone cortisol levels rocketing. This increases your chances of gaining yet more tummy fat.

Thirdly, the quality of your sleep can by affected by hormonal changes, which further impacts upon the symptoms of your menopause and that dreaded belly fat. Thanks to decreased levels of the appetite suppressant leptin and increased levels of the appetite stimulant ghrelin, you are also far more likely to make poorer food choices and overeat. And when you feel your diet's not working, it can be tempting to just give up and reach for the cake.

So why doesn't it happen to everyone?

Lifestyle choices, habits, stress and nutrition all play a big part, so for some people it's easy to just carry on as they are and not gain a pound. Others notice that the lifestyle they've enjoyed for years with no negative effects can suddenly start to take its toll.

Nobody here is going to tell you that you can't enjoy your favourite foods or have to make sweeping overnight changes. But we can offer some advice and tips, and making just a few small, gradual tweaks will really start to pay off over time.

THE NATURAL APPROACH

Making positive lifestyle choices will keep you fit and healthy, too. Here's how to get started:

Reduce your stress

It's important to relax as much as possible to keep stress at bay. This means asking for help when you feel your stress levels rising. Increased cortisol can mean that you'll pile on weight and become prone to overeating, and can make you feel really rotten. Taking a leisurely walk can help too.

Know your nutrition

To keep menopausal symptoms and belly fat at bay, you need to be eating plenty of meat protein and plant-based proteins, healthy fats, fresh fruit and mineral-rich green leafy veggies. At the same time, you should think about reducing or eliminating processed grains and sugars.

A healthy mind

Stop being down on yourself, stay positive, try meditation and yoga and keep your cortisol levels down. A healthy mind can help you stay happy and keep your hormones in check at the same time.

Get more active

Just half an hour three times a week can make a big difference to our hormonal balance, blood flow, brain health and bone density. You need to get out of breath for it to be really effective, so it's time to get moving...

So as you can see, cutting calories and buying big support pants isn't the way to tackle belly fat. And neither is resigning yourself to it as part of getting older. A few lifestyle tweaks and you'll soon be feeling healthier and happier... with no belly bulge in sight.

THE MEDICAL APPROACH

Fat stored around your middle can increase your risk of heart disease and other conditions, such as diabetes.

But there's no magic pill that is going to make the fat go away. While HRT can help to reduce increasing abdominal fat after menopause – and contrary to some schools of thought is not likely to make you actually gain weight – your doctor will also want to talk to you about your lifestyle.

Your doctor can help you with nutrition and exercise tips and they – or your practice nurse – can look in more detail at your lifestyle and make some recommended adjustments. If you've been able to eat whatever you like all your life, it can be something of a shock to discover that suddenly you need to watch what you eat, but they can give you dietary and nutritional advice.

As we've described menopause as a transition, it is a good time to take stock of your life and habits, helping you to enjoy a happy and healthy life post menopause.

I'M TIRED ALL THE TIME BUT I CAN'T SLEEP. WHAT CAN I DO?

It can be so frustrating when you fall into bed exhausted and then are still lying awake hours later. And many women going through the menopause cite sleep problems as one of their biggest concerns.

Your body clock helps to regulate your sleep patterns. They are also controlled by the hormone melatonin, which helps you to feel sleepy when the sun sets. When your sleep patterns are out of whack, you need to try to regulate your body clock and your melatonin levels. HRT can also help with sleep.

Go to bed at the same time every night

It's tempting to stay up later, thinking you're more likely to drop off. But it's all about setting patterns and sticking to them – whatever day it is and wherever you are.

Step away from the smartphone!

Scrolling through social media or messages is rather addictive, but the blue light from your phone or tablet can really interfere with your sleep patterns. Try also to avoid watching television and reading e-books. It's a good idea to keep away from all these devices for a few hours before bed – again, it's about forming new habits.

Find a relaxing routine

Whatever works for you – a long bath, some yoga, writing in a journal or reading a book… whatever helps you unwind and relax before bed.

Think about your habits

Late-night coffee and alcohol can disturb your sleep, so it could be worth checking your bedtime drink. Caffeine can delay melatonin release, which actually sets your body back by up to 90 minutes.

Meanwhile, alcohol is a stimulant that can interfere with your REM (dream) cycle of sleep. Cigarettes late at night can also affect your sleep patterns. So have a look at your drinking and smoking habits and make a few adjustments until you find whatever works best for you.

UNPREDICTABLE PERIODS, AND CHANGES IN SEX DRIVE

One of the main symptoms women mention during menopause is that their periods become erratic and heavy. And one of the biggest sources of concern is vaginal dryness and loss of sex drive – in general, feeling less feminine. We'll continue our discussion of these symptoms in the following chapters.

'I started eating a plant-based diet two weeks ago and my hot flushes stopped immediately. From 10 a day to zero.'
Juliet Helps

WOMEN'S STORIES...

'When I reached the age of 45 I hadn't given menopause a second thought. Yet just six months later I had become completely consumed by it.

I hadn't felt great for a few months, nothing specific, just tired all the time and no energy, even walking my dogs had become a chore. More worryingly I had become increasingly anxious and emotional and I was struggling to cope.

Finally, my husband persuaded me to visit my doctor who took blood tests that showed I was seriously anaemic. My doctor prescribed iron tablets and told me to come back if I didn't feel better. Two weeks later I was back feeling worse, more blood tests showed a significantly raised CAI25, an indicator of, amongst other things, ovarian cancer.

Suspicious growths on my ovaries along with a large fibroid and the rapidly increasing CAI25 resulted in my gynaecologist advising a total hysterectomy including both ovaries. Hello surgical menopause!

Although I knew I was in surgical menopause, which the hot flushes confirmed, I had not been offered any advice or information at hospital and was told to go and see my GP. I was aware of HRT and had heard it was made from conjugated equine oestrogens (horse wee) and I didn't want that.

When I saw my GP I told her I didn't want HRT and that I wanted to try the natural route, she said she would prefer me to take it but supported my decision to try an alternative method. At my first appointment with the natural menopause clinic I was prescribed several herbal remedies which I was told would ease my symptoms.

A few months later things started to rapidly go downhill. My confidence evaporated overnight, I became increasingly anxious, my heart would race and I couldn't sleep at night. Each day felt darker than the last and I was dragging myself through. I became so insecure that I could not bear to be home alone during the day so my mum had to come and stay.

I felt sad, frightened and lost, I was drowning. I plucked up the shreds of my courage and called my doctor's surgery for the details of my local menopause support service, and the receptionist simply said, 'Sorry, there isn't one.' What? It seemed ridiculous, and I promised myself if I ever felt better I would take action to change this.

Soon after, my husband reached his wits' end and booked an appointment with my GP for that night. I sobbed as I told her what I'd been going through and she asked if I would consider HRT again. She then told me there was a plant-based body-identical alternative. Initially I breathed a huge sigh of relief but later I would question why nobody had ever offered me the choices before.

Just a few days later I started to feel like my old self again. This continued for several months, until I started to become anxious again, struggling to sleep. I did some research and the evidence pointed towards a lack of progesterone. As somebody who had been diagnosed with severe endometriosis I learnt that progesterone should have been prescribed for me.

So back to the doctors but instead of progesterone the doctor insisted I visit a heart specialist. I knew it wasn't a heart problem and after two wasted appointments my heart was given a clean bill of health but I was still struggling. I went back to the GP again but was told progesterone could not be prescribed to a woman who'd had a hysterectomy. Next stop was an appointment with an NHS menopause clinic four months later. When the sleep-deprived day of the consultation arrived, the doctor dismissed progesterone as a horrible hormone and suggested my doctor prescribe testosterone.

I was getting desperate so contacted a clinician-led menopause website, within a few days I had a reply to my email advising that I absolutely should have been prescribed progesterone. I took this reply to my doctor and finally received my first prescription for progesterone, almost three years after my surgery. Within days my sleep and anxiety had improved and the heart palpitations had disappeared.

The events of the last four years have changed my life, my own experience has made me realise just how much there is to do to improve menopause care and awareness. I wanted to have professional clinical knowledge so attended nurse training on menopause.

I have kept the promise I made to myself and have now created the support service that I needed, offering support, advice and information to women and their families.'

Diane Danzebrink

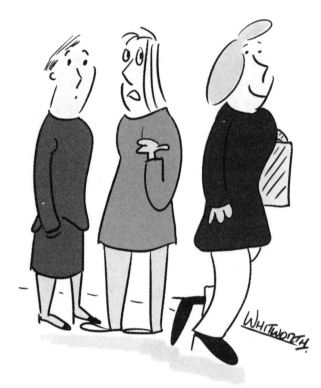

"SHE MUST BE POST-MENOPAUSAL, THAT'S THE THIRD PAIR OF WHITE JEANS SHE'S BOUGHT THIS WEEK."

4

....

How will my periods be affected?

*'I've always kept myself very fit through sport, and am aware
of my body and its changes. I had flooding, night sweats
(still have those) and I'm told mood swings (seemed fine
to me!). Running and walking helped, I'm sure. Crying
happened, but so what? My mother was of the stiff upper lip
generation and I reckon I'm the same. I don't understand
why it has to be medicalised, maybe I'm just lucky.'*
Helen Williams

In our survey, one of the top answers to what would be
the best thing about being postmenopausal was 'no more
periods', so that's something many of us will look forward to as
we approach menopause. But it's not always as straightforward
as that. Your periods probably won't just stop. Your body is in a
time of great flux, and it's a gradual process, which helps you to
recalibrate before you welcome in a period-free world. Hurray!

Over the years, you've probably come to know your periods inside out. You know how long your cycle is, how heavy your flow is, how long your period lasts and how you'll feel before, during and after. You know what's normal for you. So what can you expect and when should you seek expert help?

When the perimenopause arrives, things can seem to go a bit haywire. You might notice your once-regular period starts to become more erratic. Where your period used to last five days, now it's anything from three days to ten days and counting. Not only can this be exhausting, it's inconvenient and can be unpleasant.

WHAT COULD HAPPEN?

Nobody knows how perimenopause will affect them until it happens. But as a general guide:

• Some women find they have their normal periods right through perimenopause, then they simply stop and they never have another. This is quite unusual, however.
• Sometimes periods can stop as a result of a major life event, such as a bereavement, or a serious illness. And then never start again.
• The majority of women will experience changes from their normal periods, whether that's an increasing level of flow, longer or shorter periods or even spotting in between.

WHY DOES THIS HAPPEN?

The menopause is a time of great change for our reproductive systems. And with our hormones finding a new balance, inevitably our periods can change before they eventually disappear.

Your period is largely brought on by egg production. Oestrogen sends a signal to tell the womb lining to grow, then progesterone tells it to stop growing and prepare to receive the fertilised egg. If the egg isn't fertilised, the lining of the womb falls away as a period.

When you start to miss periods, it's because you're not making eggs. Sometimes your womb lining keeps on getting thicker and thicker (under the influence of oestrogen), and it may get so thick that it just needs to bleed, even if there's no egg there.

Missing periods, then having heavy periods because your womb lining is so thick is not at all uncommon.

CAN I GET PREGNANT WHILE I'M IN PERIMENOPAUSE?

This was another big question from women confused about the possibility of pregnancy in perimenopause and menopause. And the answer is yes, you can get pregnant in perimenopause, so it is very important to continue using contraception until after your periods have completely finished. And even then, you will need to consider protection from sexually transmitted diseases.

Did you know that in the UK more than 20 women a year over the age of 50 have a termination? It's a rather startling figure, but unintended pregnancy really does happen in this age group. While it's true that some women do choose to become pregnant a little later in life, for those who have already completed their families or chosen not to have children, this is a very big issue.

If you miss a period, don't just assume it's a sign of menopause – take a pregnancy test. And if you miss a period – or more likely, you miss several – then don't assume that you're not still ovulating. Also, remember that HRT is not a contraceptive.

Women on HRT sometimes find it hard to know when they've reached menopause, as they will still be getting artificial bleeds, just like women get periods on the pill. You can find out by stopping your HRT for a month and then having a blood test to find out if you're in the postmenopausal range. If so, you should still use contraception for another year. If not, then you can repeat the same exercise a year later. This also applies if you have a hormone coil fitted or are taking the birth control pill, as it can be difficult to know if you're still getting natural periods.

So yes, you can get pregnant while you're menopausal and yes, you can get pregnant on HRT. Be warned! So it's important to take contraception for two years following your last period if you're under 50 and one year from your last period if you're over 50.

I THOUGHT MY PERIODS HAD FINISHED, BUT I'VE SUDDENLY STARTED BLEEDING AGAIN. SHOULD I BE WORRIED?

Sometimes your ovaries can have a final flutter. Our hormones and well-being are very much connected, and sometimes an emotional life event, such as your child getting married, can affect your hormones and you might notice you start bleeding again.

Essentially, a period should be a discreet entity lasting about seven days. If you thought your periods had finished and you suddenly notice you are bleeding then you should see your doctor who may arrange for some investigations. Any bleeding which occurs more than a year after your last obvious period should be checked out by a doctor.

MY PERIODS ARE SO HEAVY, IS THERE ANYTHING I CAN DO?

Heavy periods can blight your life, especially if they drag on for what feels like forever. They can also make you anaemic. As egg release becomes less reliable, period rhythm disappears. Sometimes you enter what is called an anovulatory cycle, where an egg doesn't release at all, and then when the bleeds are further apart the prolonged, heavy bleeding women frequently complain of during the perimenopause can happen.

Women often feel they have to just put up with heavy bleeding, but when it affects your quality of life this simply isn't the case. It is certainly worth taking action if you're suffering.

So while your hormones are topsy-turvy, you don't need to sit on the sidelines and watch. There are some – often simple – tactics you can employ to help ease the transition.

THE MEDICAL APPROACH

We discuss in chapter 11 how you can get the best from your GP appointment. It is often a case of going in armed with information and prepared to ask for what you think you need, while also listening to your doctor's professional advice. Nobody should be sent away and told it's just 'their time of life'.

Your GP can sometimes prescribe progestogen tablets, which usually work to halt the bleeding immediately. Some women are referred for a trans-vaginal scan, to establish if there is any underlying cause such as a fibroid or polyp – which may be the case with younger women.

Having a Mirena coil fitted can also slow or stop your bleeding, as it tells the uterus to ignore what the ovaries are doing and stops the lining of the womb building up. It's a small, plastic device that's inserted into your womb and releases progestogen directly where it's needed and will usually stop bleeding altogether. It is also an excellent form of contraception (although please bear in mind it will protect against pregnancy but not sexually transmitted diseases).

It can stay in place for five years, and as it releases progestogen some women use this as the progestogen element of their HRT, taking oestrogen tablets or using an oestrogen patch or gel separately.

The Mirena coil is suitable for most women. If you think you'd like to have one fitted, speak to your GP or practice nurse.

Some types of HRT can also help with reducing the heavy and irregular bleeding – again, speak to your doctor. It may be necessary to make sure there isn't some other underlying cause of erratic bleeding before starting treatment, perhaps by having an ultrasound scan.

WOMEN'S STORIES...

'My mum didn't talk about the menopause. I don't remember her going through it or having symptoms. I know that she never took HRT but knew of her friends who did.

I never heard anything about my maternal grandmother's experiences, other than according to mum, "you just had to get on with it."

My first realisation of the change was when I was on an Egyptian cruise, on a day trip to Jordan, and I flooded. This had happened once or twice before but when I was due for a period.

This one took me by surprise, I was not prepared. I had to somehow find a chemist where they spoke little English. Luckily, we found a chemist where a young woman was behind a screen. With lots of eye contact and pointing she understood what I needed and I made my purchase.

I had flooded through my clothes, underwear and jeans – luckily they were black – and I used my husband's jumper to tie around my waist to disguise the bloodstain. What an uncomfortable, embarrassing afternoon I spent. I would be in my early 40s at the time.

As the months passed the flooding and irregular periods continued, the flooding got worse and worse. This is also where the hot sweats started, more like a flush for a couple of minutes at a time. I went to the doctor about the flooding, at the time I didn't know it was, or could be, the menopause.

The doctor suggested the Mirena coil containing hormones to regulate the periods, but menopause was not mentioned. The village surgery I attended did not have the facilities to fit the coil and the nearest hospital to us was more than 20 miles away. As this was something which had to be planned due to working etc, I never got around to having it done.

A few months later the flooding stopped – I probably put up with it for a couple of years. I used incontinence pads and when Tena pants came in they were a godsend. I could wear them day and night without bleeding onto the bedding or furniture. Periods slowed down to a light period for about another 12 months, and the other symptoms had started by now.'

Jane Taylor

What happens to my bones and ligaments during menopause?

'In the early 1900s, many women didn't live long beyond their menopause, it was seen as the beginning of the end. In modern times, when 60 is the new 40, it is simply the next stage. It is however the one thing that unites all women and, as such, we should discuss it and share our knowledge and feelings with each other and let it bring us closer together.'
Jo Martin

Bones are fascinating and much more than just scaffolding. Rather than being white, rigid and solid, these amazing structures are raw pink and awash with blood vessels. Their rich marrow is a lattice of fine hollow webbing to transmit stress and allow free, light movement, and is the place where our blood cells are born.

They are also hormonal powerhouses producing, among other hormones, osteocalcin, which regulates the density of calcium in our bones, and consequently their strength. Interestingly, osteocalcin also plays a role in regulating obesity and glucose tolerance. So having healthy bones, believe it or not, contributes in a truly holistic way to our positive self-esteem.

A WORD FROM A PHYSIOTHERAPIST...

Our self-image is important. It can affect our confidence, attitudes, identity and outlook on life.

While the medical world treats our body as a separate entity, our brain-body connection is a fundamental part of the way we see ourselves and the world. As our body changes, so do our attitudes towards it.

This chapter will explain what is going on with your physical tissue – bones, muscles and ligaments throughout your body, including the secretive bowl of your pelvis and sexual organs – and why it is so crucially important for our long-term health to understand and take care of them.

Women tend to have a closer relationship with their body than men, but it is not all for the better. Wrestling with our self-image in our teens, we perhaps find confidence in our later years, or maybe we just learn over time to hide our doubts better.

Childbirth is the ultimate physical challenge for the female body and its hormonal symphony, but with it comes change, consequence, confusion.

Age might bring once more those feelings of insecurity. Will I still be sexy, will I put on weight, will I become frail?

Perhaps the menopause will bring new questions to your door you never knew were coming:

Will I get osteoporosis?

Have I got a prolapse?

Why can't I make it to the loo on time?

Why can't I seem to stand up straight anymore?

And, the overarching question inside us all: Is my body turning on me?

Though many of the changes are less obvious than hot flushes and erratic periods, the physical changes are what ultimately define our progress from middle to old age.

This chapter is about how we can take control of our bodies, and begin a new generation that challenges the concept of the Old Woman.

WHAT HAPPENS TO MY BONES DURING MENOPAUSE?

The essential thing to know about bones is that their growth and health respond to load. Their sense of where pressure is coming from determines where they add density or where they break down bone tissue because it is not needed.

Hormonal changes during the menopause can affect absorption and production of calcium, which in turn affects the density and integrity of your bones. They can become weaker, leading to osteoporosis developing, which is more prevalent in women than men and suffered by over two million women in the UK today. Risk factors are linked to hormonal changes during the menopause, certain medications, as well as lifestyle factors such as smoking, drinking, or low activity levels.

Often the first sign of osteoporosis (which literally means 'porous bones') is sustaining a 'fragility fracture' – a significant fracture after falling from standing height or even less. We can also have small fractures in our spines without knowing it. This contributes to the traditional hunched posture depiction of older women, and can be the cause of the 'dowager hump', though this can also be just stiffness and poor posture. Posture is also about a lot more than just how we look – a bent spine will reduce the available space for our lungs, restrict our movement and blood flow and compress our organs.

WHAT DOES THE FUTURE HOLD?

It is clear that our bodies lose muscle bulk, nerve endings and bone density as we age. Our tissues tend to get stiffer at a cellular level and our collagen production slows.

As we get older, we tend to move around less overall and reduce our resistance or high-impact activity. Quite reasonably, our bones therefore decide they have less use and quietly go about reducing their density and strength, as it is not efficient to maintain this tissue if we aren't going to use it.

Our spinal ligaments, held for many hours a day in a forward curved position, will lengthen with this load and over time lose their elasticity and remain irreversibly long. Other ligaments, such as those wrapped around our hip joints, gradually stiffen if we don't make a conscious effort to open up our bodies and stretch out.

Our soft tissues (skin and muscle) replace cells more slowly as time goes on and as they lose the stimulation that makes them grow and regenerate. Internal connective tissue becomes more fibrous and less elastic, repairing more slowly after any damage. These changes take place over decades, and are already starting to happen by our mid-30s.

WHAT CAN I DO?

Ageing is an individual experience, and 'just getting old' should never be the defining factor of what happens to you. Your attitude and lifestyle are arguably the most important factors in what cards the years will deal you.

And while you can't stop the ageing process, there's plenty you can do to help yourself. You can't undo wrinkles, but you can keep your skin healthy by preventing further damage from the sun, for example. You can grow muscle, improve bone density, generate millions more brain neurons, at whatever age, whatever stage of life.

But how?

There are some lifestyle tweaks you can make that can help:

Caffeine and cola drinks containing phosphoric acid have long been associated with decreased bone density as they increase calcium excretion by actually stimulating bone breakdown, and at the other end of things can affect calcium absorption in the gut.

Smoking is a universal risk factor for poor healing of bones and tissues. If you just love your cola for energy or find a ciggie is the best way to calm you down, it could be time to take a look at your lifestyle, to avoid far more severe problems in the long term.

The same goes for your muscles. Sit all day? Your bottom will start to sag. Hunch at your computer? Your shoulder muscles will ache – but they will also get bigger to cope with the load you are asking them to burden. This exacerbates poor posture and altered body shape that is hard to reverse.

Get physically active. Aside from all the psychological benefits of exercise, the physical benefits are quite staggering.

STANDING STRONG

- Can you get up off the floor?
- Can you stand up out of a chair – hands free?
- Can you go up stairs without holding on to a banister?

These may seem ridiculous questions, but just try. You may be surprised by the habits our world of convenience has got us into. Do you need to grab furniture for help? Do you make that 'floof' noise as the effort puffs you out? Do you have a strategy if you fell with no one there to help? If you find these things difficult to do now, you will be putting yourself into a high-risk falls category in later life.

Some of us have elderly parents, and have experienced at first hand the shock of once-strong characters being weakened physically and psychologically before our eyes. Falls are one of the major reasons for admission to care homes, but of course they happen at any age. A small slip or overbalance could literally be a life-changing moment, and it's worth preparing for.

What kind of exercise is important? Research shows that to improve bone strength as well as muscle power and endurance, it really is resistance work, i.e. weights, that will make the difference to your body.

If you are a sworn enemy of exercise, it's time to wave the white flag: strength and basic agility is your ally for the rest of your life.

WHAT SORT OF ACTIVITY IS BEST?

Never fear, it doesn't have to mean 100 press-ups by dawn. It's a series of small choices that you can make every day.

- You've probably heard it before, but take the stairs. Run up them if circumstances allow – always make sure you're safe.
- Push up out of your chair with your legs and bottom, don't haul up using your arms.
- Squat correctly to pick things up. Keep your back straight and feet at least hip-width apart.
- Walk, don't drive, wherever possible.

Every time you make these choices, you are building a strong future for your skeleton and your independence. Moving more may not seem important... until we can't.

WON'T EXERCISING MAKE MY MUSCLES BULKY?

Like the myth that eating low fat will make you thin (it doesn't), it is also incorrect that building muscle will 'bulk' you up. In fact, 5lb of fatty tissue takes up many times more space than 5lb of muscle, which means you will get slimmer, not bigger.

And here's the great bit about it: muscle will burn calories while you sleep or while you sit people-watching at a wine bar in the summer. Toned muscles and strong bones will only ever improve your posture, your endurance and your confidence. That is not to say that cardio exercise doesn't have its benefits – your heart and lungs are so important to keep healthy. But try doing 20 squats… you'll soon realise that this is not just weight training but cardiovascular exercise at the same time, and at its most challenging.

Cardiovascular exercise is great for boosting your metabolism and is certainly beneficial for daily activity. However, cardio is simply burning off your last meal and helping to process the next. Resistance training addresses the deeper metabolic balance of the body, altering your body composition for the better. If you're perimenopausal, you do need to build up your calcium reserves, and the right kind of resistance training can help you do this.

There are a thousand gyms to join with free-weights areas, but the best weights training is with your own body weight, and in the natural environment. It's a perfect, proportional strength for each individual to have and to move their way through life. It also means you aren't just training one muscle at a time, flexing your biceps or hamstrings repeatedly in one plane of movement.

Our muscles are layered throughout our bodies in diagonals and spirals, for twisting, turning, reaching. So when choosing a fitness programme, look for a system that incorporates natural three-dimensional movement, that focuses on multiple muscle activation, that challenges your strength, not just gets you out of breath. Like these:

Yoga is fantastic for this kind of movement, as there are lots of poses that incorporate rotation and encourage you to move through full range. This is also great for strength because moving from pose to pose and holding postures can really be challenging for your muscles.

Swimming is also brilliant resistance work and front crawl allows for both long diagonal movements as well as challenging your mid-section to stabilise you in the water. For more dynamic work, consider **boxing** (great for stress relief!) as a punch should come all the way from the foot with correct technique!

Or if that sounds like too much for your energy levels, some types of **dancing**, such as salsa, are brilliant for core work, balance, getting moderately out of breath and having a lot of fun.

YOU HAVE CONTROL

The amazing thing about our physical body is that we have the power to change it. We can make great gains in just a few short months. Hormones can be very mysterious but the physical body, although intertwined with these, is refreshingly straightforward once you clear out all the myths.

USE IT OR LOSE IT

Though it may sound a little firm and forthright, this is the truth of it. There's no need for any gimmick, restrictive diet, or bizarre regime for a long-lasting, healthy relationship with your body.

Connect with your body as an ally, not an enemy.

'Menopause for me has been a far more positive experience than I was expecting. I had particularly difficult periods and felt that I was a slave to my hormones. Menopause has been very liberating. Whilst I have got several symptoms (crashing fatigue, muscle fatigue and aches, temperature changes) they don't bother me as much as my periods. I feel more content, calmer and I don't feel like I am on a hormonal rollercoaster.'
Kathryn

WOMEN'S STORIES...

'Recently menopause kicked in big time for me. While I had some over-heating moments, the worst thing about it was that I felt completely exhausted all the time.

And on top of the fatigue I felt irritable, vulnerable and emotionally on the edge.

After two tearful visits to the GP to seek reassurance that I wasn't going crazy, a moment of insight occurred while I was out walking with the dog. Here I was going through all this and what was the point of it anyway, every month of my adult life I'd had a menstrual cycle. Now this was at an end and my body was going through another transition, and for what... I DON'T HAVE CHILDREN!

And then the penny dropped... here it was again... that sadness about not being a mum. I thought I'd dealt with this, had moved on and accepted it but I was wrong. Here was another stage in my journey.

Being childless is a silent, intangible and invisible grief that can make you feel very alone. It has the same emotions of other bereavements but it's about grieving what's not to be rather than grieving what you've treasured and lost.

Recognising that this sadness was creating a deeper dimension to my symptoms was a turning point for me. I now knew what I was dealing with – loss.

Realising that loss was a recurring theme in my life, I decided to have some therapy specifically to clear the emotion of grief. With this support, I was able to realise my grief had become a barrier, something I had been holding on to. It was quite literally keeping me stuck. This new insight helped me to let it go.

And since investing in myself in this way, things have changed enormously for me. My energy is much improved, I feel more connected in my relationships, and my menopausal symptoms have mostly gone.

And I now recognise that I am not on my own. I have a supportive personal network around me, which includes my family and two close friends who are both childless and who listen to me and get who I am. I also have a network based on playing tennis, socially and competitively.

Being active and doing the things that give me joy, such as playing tennis and walking the dog, also keep me strong and positive.

So, all in all life is in better flow for me now. Menopause helped me to acknowledge and face a painful truth and feel all the stronger for it.'

Sally Coombs

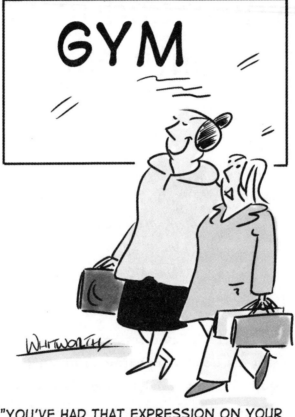

"YOU'VE HAD THAT EXPRESSION ON YOUR FACE EVER SINCE YOU STARTED DOING THOSE KEGEL EXERCISES."

What is vaginal dryness and urinary incontinence?

'For me, the vaginal dryness has been the worst and most painful thing ever. I went to the doctor's about it, but menopause was not mentioned. I was given something to insert on an applicator.'
Jane Taylor

Vaginal dryness is another aspect of menopause, and one that can be quite upsetting or distressing if you are suffering badly. You're not going to suddenly 'dry up' overnight, but your vagina needs hormones to stay supple, so as your hormone levels dip you can notice that you are less naturally lubricated.

While you might feel comfortable talking to your doctor about your hot flushes and night sweats, you may not feel the same when talking about your dry vagina! Understandably,

many women are embarrassed and don't realise how common vaginal dryness is.

Some women also worry about suffering from incontinence as they go through menopause. You might find yourself getting up more in the night, and urinary tract infections are more common in menopausal women because vaginal dryness is caused by low oestrogen, and other genital tissues, including your urinary tract, can be affected.

In this chapter, we'll look at what vaginal dryness is, what causes it and what you can do about it. We'll also examine the different types of incontinence and explore the treatments.

WHAT IS VAGINAL DRYNESS?

As the amount of oestrogen reduces in your body during the menopause, your vagina becomes less lubricated and stretchy. Using chemical products such as medicated wipes, sprays or even some types of washing powder can also lead to vaginal dryness.

Vaginal dryness or atrophy is also called atrophic vaginitis. Some doctors refer to it as Genitourinary Syndrome of the Menopause (GSM), as it is not just your vagina that is affected. The low levels of oestrogen in your body can lead to thinning and weakening of the tissues around the neck of your bladder, or around the opening for urine to pass (the urethra). For example, urinary symptoms that may occur include an urgency to get to the toilet and recurring urinary infections or cystitis.

Oestrogen is important in that it acts as a natural lubricant in your vagina and helps to keep this area healthy and moist. Oestrogen also stimulates the cells that line your vagina to produce glycogen. Glycogen is a compound that encourages the presence of helpful germs (bacteria) that protect your vagina from infections.

This lack of oestrogen tends to cause the tissues around your vagina to become thinner, dryer and inflamed. These changes can take months or even years to develop and vary between women.

Your vagina may shrink a little and expand less easily during sex, making sexual intercourse more painful or uncomfortable. Your vulva may become thin, dry and itchy. You may notice that your vulva or vagina has become red and sore. You may also find you have episodes of thrush more frequently. Many women have symptoms of vaginal pain and discomfort throughout the day, so it is often not just a problem to those women who are sexually active.

As the skin around your vagina becomes more sensitive, it is then more likely to itch. This can make you prone to scratching, which in turn makes you even more inclined to itch, and so on.

All these symptoms can be present long after your menopause, even when you don't have any other symptoms. They are very common symptoms that affect the vast majority of women at some time after the menopause. You are also more likely to experience symptoms as more years pass after your menopause. They occur in at least seven out of ten women after the menopause and can occur even if you are taking HRT.

The good news is there are some really effective treatments available from your GP, and lubricants and moisturisers can also help.

THE MEDICAL APPROACH

The usual treatment is replacing the oestrogen in your vagina and the surrounding tissues. A cream, vaginal tablet or ring containing oestrogen is often prescribed and they work really well. A vaginal tablet is a very small tablet that you insert into your vagina with a small applicator. The vaginal tablets and creams are usually used every day for two weeks, and then used twice a week thereafter. The ring is soft and flexible with a centre that contains the oestrogen hormone. This ring releases a steady, low dose of oestrogen each day and it lasts for three months. It can be inserted and replaced easily by yourself, or by your nurse or doctor.

Using topical oestrogen in this way is not the same as taking HRT as it is not absorbed into your body. This is because these preparations work to restore oestrogen to your vagina and surrounding tissues without giving oestrogen to your whole body. These preparations can be safely used by most women and can also be used on a regular basis over a long period of time (usually indefinitely) as your symptoms will often return if you stop this treatment.

Taking HRT systemically can also improve symptoms of vaginal dryness. However, some women who take HRT also need these local treatments to relieve these symptoms. It is completely safe to have vaginal oestrogen with HRT.

Your symptoms should improve after about three months of treatment. You should see your doctor if your symptoms don't improve, as they can sometimes be due to other conditions. It is also very important to see your doctor if you have any unusual bleeding from your vagina if you are receiving hormone treatment.

THE NATURAL APPROACH

Vaginal lubricants and moisturisers can be used either with hormones or on their own and are usually also very effective. These are available either from your doctor or to buy from various chemists or online. There are many different products available and it is important that you find one that suits you.

Moisturisers are used regularly, whereas lubricants are usually used during sexual intercourse.

Some lubricants actually contain irritating ingredients like glycerin and glycols. The pH of the lubricant is also important, because if a lubricant is too alkaline it can also lead to urinary tract infections, thrush or bacterial vaginosis. Check on the packet to find a product that is pH balanced, ideally between 3.8pH and 4.5pH, and which lists the ingredients.

Do a skin test before putting the product on – there is nothing worse than a stinging, burning or itching vulva and vagina. It is best to avoid any products that stimulate, warm or cool as they often contain ingredients you find in chillies and menthol that are not good for vaginal health. Flavoured lubricants contain glycerin and sweeteners, too.

If you find a product irritates, you should stop using it and try another variety, as ingredients in each product can be very different.

Some women use KY jelly but although this is what some doctors use when examining a woman, it is not an effective lubricant for vaginal dryness.

Every woman is different and so it is very important to find a product that works for you. Vaginal moisturisers and lubricants can be used alongside vaginal oestrogens. It is usually advisable to use them at slightly different times, though.

It's important to note that oil-based lubricants are not suitable for use with condoms.

WILL I BECOME INCONTINENT?

Urinary incontinence is very common and affects many women in different ways. You may find that you leak urine if you jump or sneeze or you might notice that you can't hold on to urine for as long as you used to be able to. Urinary incontinence is often not really spoken about, which is a shame because there are some really effective treatments available for women. Urinary incontinence is more common during and after the menopause.

There are two types of urinary incontinence: stress incontinence and urge incontinence. Some women have a combination of stress and urge incontinence.

Stress incontinence occurs when you can't hold on to as much urine as before so you're more likely to leak urine when you cough or sneeze, and this is usually due to the muscles and tissues that support your bladder becoming weaker with time. Many factors contribute to this and include having children, being constipated, if you are overweight or obese, and having reduced muscle tone, which is associated with low levels of oestrogen in the menopause. Having a weak pelvic floor, the muscles and tissues that support your bladder, contributes to this.

Urge incontinence is when you can't hold on to as much urine as before so you need to rush to the toilet quicker than you used to. You may notice that you don't get much warning before you need to go to the toilet either. In addition, you may find you have to get up more often at night to pass urine.

Urge incontinence can be caused by infection, destruction of the nerves controlling your bladder or thinning of the tissues of the tubing along which your urine flows.

Urge incontinence is usually due to an overactive bladder. This means that your bladder does not fill up properly and tells your brain that you need to empty it even when it's not full. You may find that you need to pass urine more frequently when you are stressed.

THE MEDICAL APPROACH

Vaginal ring pessaries that work to support your internal organs are available to combat stress incontinence. They can work really well and are usually replaced every 6-12 months. You can still have sexual intercourse with them in place.

The oestrogen in HRT can also help this kind of incontinence in the way that it helps all other muscles, by improving your muscle tone.

Having low levels of oestrogen, which occurs as you go through the menopause, can also affect the lining of your bladder and your urethra so will often contribute to and worsen the symptoms of urge incontinence.

If the following simple measures are not effective, there are different types of medication that can work really well. If one type of medication does not work for you, you may be offered an alternative that is effective.

If medication does not help, there are different operations that may be offered to you, depending on the cause and severity of your symptoms.

THE NATURAL APPROACH

If you've had children, you'll probably have been told (a lot) about the importance of doing your pelvic floor exercises after the birth. But quite often, as the years pass, we forget all about it and it's only as we get older and maybe start to show signs of bladder leakage that we suddenly realise all those Kegels we used to do have been long forgotten. It's important to note, too, that if you haven't had children you will still really benefit from doing pelvic floor exercises.

The good news is that just one simple breathing technique can help you correct your muscle tone, recover from trauma, improve your sexual function and stop bladder leakage, and is great for tackling stress incontinence.

Your pelvic floor is a large web of muscles that runs from your tailbone right around to your pubic bone and across your hip bones. Its functions include supporting all of your internal organs, maintaining your continence and also helping you to enjoy sexual sensation and orgasm. Pelvic floor dysfunction is usually caused by childbirth, being overweight or over-stressed, and hormonal changes in menopause can weaken the muscles and tissues in this area.

Breathing correctly is vital when it comes to pelvic floor health. It helps to relax any muscles we are tensing, including those in the diaphragm or pelvic floor. In turn, this helps to lower the levels of the stress hormone cortisol, rebalance your sex hormones, alleviate menopause symptoms and make you feel calmer.

To enjoy maximum benefits, practise this exercise twice a day for around five minutes each time. Find somewhere quiet to sit where you won't be disturbed.

1. Settle comfortably and gently close your eyes.
2. Bring your attention to your breath, inhaling through your nose and exhaling through your mouth.
3. Breathe right down into your belly. Imagine that your abdomin is a balloon that inflates as you breathe in and shrinks as you breathe out. The chest should only move a little as your tummy is doing most of the movement.
4. Inhale for a count of four and then exhale for a count of eight. This extended exhale is the perfect way to kick-start whole body relaxation and feel calmer and more connected to your body.

The good news is that by practising this simple breathing exercise, you can activate those pelvic floor muscles and help improve your pelvic floor.

If you believe you might be suffering from pelvic floor dysfunction, please see your GP so you can get an accurate diagnosis.

While this breathing technique is great for stress incontinence, if you suffer from urge incontinence you could try cutting out drinks containing caffeine, such as coffee and cola. These can irritate the lining of your bladder and make urge incontinence worse. Other drinks such as fruit juices can also irritate your bladder.

Although reducing or even stopping caffeine intake is very important, you still need to drink plenty of fluids. If you do not drink enough fluids such as water, your body makes concentrated urine and this can irritate the lining of your bladder, which will often make your symptoms worse.

A WORD FROM A PHYSIOTHERAPIST...

Though it's embarrassing, this subject is so important to address, as our bladders and bowels are as fundamental to good health and longevity as our brain and lungs.

Even though the body bravely holds up and copes on the 'odd' occasion, as we age the integrity of our tissues decreases, and symptoms can suddenly start to appear far more regularly, even when we are not changing our usual habits.

Moving beyond Kegels

Kegel exercises – squeezing the pelvic floor muscles – can help improve symptoms. However, there are lots of limitations to these – not least that the pelvic floor muscles, which support the bladder and uterus, are quite difficult to access and many women really aren't sure whether they are squeezing the right bits.

Things are further complicated by the fact that the pelvic floor doesn't act alone, and weakness elsewhere, such as in our bottoms or abdomen or scar tissue, can interfere with its activation and tone.

The pelvic floor can even be *too* strong – causing issues such as constipation, back pain, and even dryness and pain during sex. If you have religiously done Kegels and your symptoms haven't changed, then it may be time to try something different.

What can you do for yourself?

This is tricky, as without an elaborate angling of mirrors and knowing what you are really feeling when you feel it, it's easy to go off on a tangent. But there are some easy things you can do to narrow down your specific problem and start to tackle it.

Take stock

Do you ever leak urine during activities such as lifting, running or simply laughing? This is called stress incontinence and is the most common form of continence dysfunction. Though it's possible to manage these 'accidents' socially, it can quickly reduce women's fitness, bladder control and confidence if left unchecked. Try making a note of when it happens over a couple of weeks and you will start to build a picture of how big a problem this really is for you.

How often do you have to go to the loo each day?

Somewhere between five and seven times is 'normal', with one visit to the bathroom at night at most. If you're going more often than this, or if you realise you've started to reduce your fluid intake to avoid going so often, then you're exhibiting patterns of potential 'urge incontinence'.

Take a peek

Though many women may balk at this suggestion, one of the most important facets of any physical rehabilitation is to improve your relationship with your body, so you feel more like a 'team' rather than fighting yourself through embarrassment or fear.

Some may not have wanted to look 'down there' since their last labour, but there is wondrous variety in what we look like, and your own body is nothing to be scared of, even if it has changed over time.

On the more internal folds of tissue, you should look slightly moist and be a warm pink colour, similar to the inside of your mouth. If you are particularly pale, dry, or overly red or sore looking, these are signs that you may need some specialist guidance to restore your genital health.

Try giving a cough while you are looking at yourself in the mirror

Does anything suddenly bulge outwards as the pressure peaks? Do you even leak a little? Or does everything appear to tighten and lift? Leaking or bulging is a sign that the pelvic floor isn't activating as well as it needs to.

Do a Kegel as you normally would. What do you see happening? Does it look like everything is pushing downwards, or lifting up? Do you notice your bottom squeezing hard, but not much else happening? Does your tummy pull in or outwards as you tense?

Correct Kegels result in a lifting of the undercarriage upwards into the pelvis. Any bulging, or tensing of the bottom or pushing out of your tummy means that your brain and the pelvic floor have a bit more communicating to do before you are nailing those sets and reps safely and correctly.

Light at the end of the tunnel

The good news is there really is something you can do about it. Not just the Kegels, but simpler things – improving posture and strength, even learning how to relax.

You can strengthen your pelvic floor at any age, learn to manage leaky moments, ease long-held scar tissue and get back in control of your toilet habits. And there are specialists out there who can identify your individual issues and help make a plan for change.

Simply finding out what information, local specialists, contraptions and solutions there are out there may make you feel more empowered… and even perhaps more happy to talk and share your experiences. You are not alone.

WOMEN'S STORIES...

'It's not something widely talked about, but women's intimate health during and after the menopause is an important topic. By understanding and properly caring for the delicate vaginal and vulval environment, uncomfortable symptoms can be avoided, and a general sense of enhanced sexual health and well-being can be experienced.

Low libido in postmenopausal women and the call for testosterone therapy on the NHS has been covered in the press, but vaginal dryness, one of the most common symptoms of menopause, is under-treated due to embarrassment and is seldom openly discussed.

In these days of social media obsession, where we share so much with our friends, how sad it is that we don't talk about this issue, which can have such a huge impact on our lives.

When I reached menopausal age I thought back to a holiday I had with my parents in the USA when my mother must have been about 51 years old. I remember her wanting to open the window as we sped down the highways because she was too hot. She also dashed into air-conditioned shops in New York whenever a hot flush rendered her into a soggy mess, but she didn't talk to me about this from that day onwards.

When I started to experience some perimenopausal urinary symptoms, my urologist never suggested that they might be related to oestrogen depletion – I had to discover that for myself and only when I found a sympathetic urogynaecologist was the link between lack of oestrogen, vaginal dryness and urinary symptoms fully explained.

My very sensitive, patient and loving husband was as surprised as I was at the symptoms that I was experiencing. He is now extremely knowledgeable about all female intimate health issues but still says that "menopausal vaginal dryness is the best kept secret after Father Christmas" – sadly the revelation, when it comes, is a lot less pleasant than the stocking at the end of the bed!

We need to talk to our daughters as they approach menopause and we need to talk to our friends, and our partners need to talk to their friends, too. There is help but you may need to go to your doctor with a clear idea of how you want to approach the challenge of dealing with the symptoms of menopause. There are plenty of natural solutions and organic lubricants and moisturisers can help with vaginal dryness on a daily basis and make sex more comfortable without compromising vaginal health with potentially harmful chemical ingredients.'

Lavinia Winch

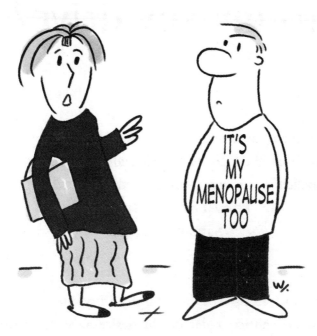

"I KNOW WE TALKED ABOUT
YOU BEING SUPPORTIVE..."

7

....

What will happen to my sex drive?

*'I made being perimenopausal a good thing – it's given me
a new lease of life. I don't care what anyone thinks of me and
I'm more willing to take control of situations when previously
I would have stayed quiet.'*
Samantha Evans

Libido, or sex drive, differs hugely in women anyway, but you may notice a decline in desire as your menopause approaches. Post menopause, some women find the cessation of their periods liberating, while others find sex just isn't high on their agenda any more.

After years of adult life, most people find a realistic balance between the demands of a busy life and a healthy sex life (which is different for everybody), but the possible effects of the menopause can take their toll on inclination and confidence in the bedroom. A night tossing and turning with hot flushes can kill off a desire for anything but sleep, and this easily becomes a way of life – as in so many aspects of life, 'luxuries' like sex are often put to the bottom of the priority list.

While it's easy to blame the menopause, it's also important to look at your lifestyle and personal circumstances. Perhaps you have teenage children in the house and don't feel like having sex when they're in the next room. Or maybe you have elderly parents living with you. Or a combination of both.

In this chapter, we'll explore more about what could happen to your sex drive when you're perimenopausal and beyond.

THE MEDICAL APPROACH

Midlife is often a tiring place to be – for example, if you have and are caring for growing children and elderly parents, while often still working at a hectic pace. So it's time to get realistic. What would you like from your sex life and what's inhibiting you? If you have a good, sound relationship and are generally otherwise happy, your hormones could be to blame. In this case, hormone replacement therapy (HRT) could help (see our **Managing your menopause** chapter for more information). Some women find that testosterone can really help with this issue.

If you're suffering from vaginal dryness, it could be that sex is painful, which can lead to a reduced libido (see our **What is vaginal dryness and urinary incontinence?** chapter for more information).

For some women, loss of sex drive is more in your head than in your genitals. In these cases, you could speak to an experienced psychosexual counsellor to guide you forward.

THE NATURAL APPROACH

Unless you go through an early menopause, perimenopause generally starts in our 40s and continues into our 50s. So we're experiencing the signs of ageing at the same time – more wrinkles and grey hair, fat we can't shift and feeling increasingly forgetful.

Sex can offer great stress-busting qualities, helping you disconnect from the everyday world and feel more intimate with your partner. Remember the old adage 'use it or lose it'? Well, when it comes to your sex drive it's a good one to bear in mind. Regular sexual intimacy, with a partner or solo, can keep your body responsive and improve blood flow.

If it's an emotional block that's stopping you wanting sex, keep the lines of communication open with your partner – talk to them about how you're feeling so they understand why you might not feel like being physically intimate as often as before.

Pelvic floor exercises can help. While it sometimes feels like these are mentioned all the time, they can help you stay tight and, again, keep the blood flow to the area strong. Eating healthy fats like olive oil, avocado and coconut oil can also help to keep your tissues young, firm and responsive. It's also important to include collagen in your diet, which you'll find in dark green vegetables, meat and fish.

A WORD FROM A PHYSIOTHERAPIST...

Healthy, functional sexual organs are in part the result of a combination of 'passive' support, i.e. the ligaments and fascia (connective tissue), and 'active' support, i.e. the muscles of the pelvic floor. The passive structures are there mainly to counteract gravity at rest, stabilise the organs against excessive movement, and give each structure its own space in the abdomen in relation to its neighbours.

If, for example, the uterus is removed in a hysterectomy, often the connective tissue is rearranged so the other organs and structures (intestines, bladder, vagina, etc.) don't lose their mutual support or fall into the gap left behind, leading to prolapse.

The active support of the pelvic floor muscles comes into play when we need to control our inter-abdominal pressure, such as when we stand up, cough, jump, or lift something.

The pelvic floor muscle group also has an important role in orgasm. The muscles contract at the moment of climax and this feeling can be intensified by increasing their strength. It is also important for these muscles to be able to relax to allow comfortable penetration and to be supple and flexible to allow variety of movement and positioning. Just like the male penis, the female pelvic floor receives an increased blood flow when aroused and this is crucial for the vagina to produce its natural lubrication and for the clitoris to become engorged. Nerves are very bloodthirsty structures and benefit greatly from increased blood flow to the area, heightening sensitivity to touch and pressure. Reduced muscle mass can reduce the flow of blood, the intensity of or ability to orgasm, and increase vaginal dryness.

What are the common effects of the menopause on your sexual organs?

Ageing for both men and women can increase the weakening of 'passive' supportive tissue throughout the body, including within the pelvis. Factors such as traumatic childbirths or gynaecological surgery can weaken these structures and in many cases damage to this tissue only starts to reveal itself in later life as cell regeneration slows.

To retain control of pelvic function, your 'active' muscles need to take a greater role… just when they are also experiencing changes through the menopause. Muscle density gradually reduces (at around 5 per cent per year), accelerating significantly in the postmenopausal years (up to 25 per cent per year), and requires input to maintain and improve strength, reaction-speed and endurance.

It may be at this point in your life that you first become aware of trauma sustained by your pelvic floor during childbirth, even if this was decades earlier. Any trauma to muscle will weaken it significantly in the short term, and that muscle often loses significant bulk and tone.

An episiotomy is a medical cut through the pelvic floor to allow a baby more room to pass through. If such a deep cut was applied to a bicep or thigh muscle, it would take months of active rehabilitation to return to normal function. In 'external' muscles we often work hard to strengthen and regain function, but this seems to be passed over when the muscles are less obvious to the eye. So although it is not uncommon for women to have significant weakness or loss of muscle bulk after a tear or episiotomy, they may be entirely unaware of it. Even those who are aware usually put any unusual long-term effects down to an inevitable consequence of 'just being a mum'.

The body is a wonderful thing and will find the best way to compensate for a problem without having to bother your conscious mind too much. Only when this task becomes much harder will your body start to show significant signs of struggling. So if you had major tears or trauma to your perineum during labour and received minimal, if any, rehabilitation, or have had minor continence issues since then, you may well expect to experience an acceleration of symptoms or a worsening of function during and after menopause.

In the context of sexual health, combining perhaps poor sleeping, mood swings, pain, discomfort or tightness, and dryness, it is extremely understandable for some of us to feel that the case for a healthy sex life is hopeless.

What's the answer?

There is good news! The body has a remarkable ability to regenerate and regrow tissue in most cases, except perhaps in cases of severe nerve damage that would be referred to a specialist. This is the case in the bones, the brain and the muscles. And the pelvic floor is just that – muscles that will respond to any consistent training programme designed for their improved strength and flexibility.

What you can do for yourself

Be honest

Take a few minutes to define what you think is bringing your sex life to a halt. Is it physical discomfort? Is it self-confidence taking a dive, and what exactly is it that is causing this lack of confidence? Is it everything else getting in the way? Is it a lack of desire, and is that a total lack of desire or do you find arousal in different scenarios/stimulus than you did before?

You may be surprised by what you discover – though sex is a physical activity, do not underestimate the incredibly powerful hold your brain and your mental well-being have over it. If you are stressed, this not only affects your inclination to have sex (despite it providing very effective stress relief for many) but it also alters hormone production, lubrication and enjoyment. It may not be that your sex drive has disappeared at all – perhaps it is being blocked by other factors that are taking precedence.

Get to know yourself
You may be very familiar and comfortable with how your genitals look and feel, but if not it may help you to defuse a few fears to take a look. It may also give you the clue to what you can do about certain problems.

If dryness seems to be your major problem, you may find that your vulva looks quite pale and lax rather than a warm pink colour and moist. This could be a sign of vaginal atrophy, a thinning of tissues around the vaginal area. This can sometimes result in the vagina becoming dry and sore.

Knowing what you look like will also help you identify changes as they occur as life progresses – as we know, nothing stays still for long, so it pays to keep an eye on your precious parts.

Practise, practise, practise…
Following on from familiarising yourself with your anatomy, it is definitely worth taking some time to get the body used to regular stimulation, and many find that doing this alone removes some of the pressure from doing it with a partner. Regular solo

activity will reinforce neural pathways between your brain and your sexual organs, and make them more accessible going forward.

Frequent stimulation will improve blood flow to your organs and may well help improve your natural lubrication, strength and suppleness of tissues without any need for medications. This is not particularly specialist advice – the principle of 'use it or lose it' applies to the whole body and it is common sense, a refreshingly simple approach that really can make big changes. Additionally, it is worth trying gentle stimulation with plenty of lubricant if you are feeling sore (as long as there is no infection or broken tissue).

Any increase in blood flow to the area, such as regular orgasms, will promote a faster recovery, and perhaps reassure a worried mind that everything can function well under the right conditions. Pelvic floor contractions and strengthening is also an essential component to healthy muscle maintenance and increases blood circulation of oxygen and nutrients to the area. If you feel tight and tense, masturbation may feel like too much for you, but it might be helpful to think of your pelvic floor muscles like any other muscle – they behave the same way and can benefit from similar treatment, such as stretching. You can help your muscles relax and stretch gently using your fingers and deep belly breathing. Insert a thumb or finger into the lower vagina, lubricated if necessary, take a normal breath in and then apply a slow, consistent backwards pressure to the back wall of your vagina on your exhale. Repeat three or four times and you should feel your pelvic floor start to stretch and gradually relax. Stretches generally benefit most from a 20–30 second duration, during which you may also feel muscles that you didn't know were tense, such as your bottom muscles or your chest, relax too.

Once comfortable with this practice, you can start to explore deeper into your vagina, using the same breathe-and-stretch-on-the-exhale technique. Is one side more tender than the other? More bulky or harder to the touch? Work on both sides, aiming for relaxed, supple muscles. You can also do your pelvic floor exercises while you are feeling internally – this is often a great way to discover whether you are doing them correctly. You should feel a forwards and upwards lift of the back of the vaginal wall as you contract your pelvic floor. Pressing on the side wall, you should feel the muscles push up and inwards against your finger. Again, you can compare the strength on either side to become more familiar with your individual anatomy.

Don't be disheartened if it takes more sessions than you expected to feel an improvement. You may not have been aware, but your pelvic floor might have been holding tension for many years – in fact, it is increasingly common, even in women in their 20s who have a hectic stressful lifestyle – so give it time. Again, there is no 'normal', and taking enough time for you as an individual is important – an anxious mind will naturally retain tension in the muscles.

What do you really want?

Once you are happier in yourself and your body is starting to regain normal function, you can gradually reintroduce other factors, such as a partner. If you have got to this stage with your partner already, perhaps consider going forward what you would like from your sex life. It is often different to what society would have us believe – there is no 'right' amount of sex, no 'normal' in terms of style or pace. It may also be different to what you thought you wanted, or what you used to like – so again, it may be helpful to do some self-reflection and work out what's right for you, right now.

It may be that you want to forget all about it in deference to other issues in your life; realising that and accepting it may well help you return to it with more confidence and optimism when you are ready – if you want to return at all.

> *'Life can be even better after the menopause if you have a loving relationship.'*
> Lesley Foster Wright

WOMEN'S STORIES...

'I'm 49 and perimenopausal. I had what I call my "lightbulb moment" four years ago. I had read yet another depressing menopause article in the press, talking about the inevitable weight gain, decreased libido and vaginal dryness, alongside the usual stock photo of a miserable, frumpy woman sitting on a bed.

Like many women, I really didn't identify with what was being said or the image portrayed, so I decided to make some changes as I journeyed through the perimenopause and menopause.

There are only so many years when you can use your youngest child as an excuse for your muffin top. It's okay when they're small but not when they are heading towards their teens!

My husband and I have been together for 26 years, and married for nearly 20. Like many couples, we had gained weight over the years, making us feel unhealthy and uncomfortable. Having a family history of heart disease, we both thought we should try to cut our risks, too.

After watching a television programme about the 5:2 diet, my husband was inspired. Seeing him lose weight after only two weeks, I decided to join him. I've tried slimming clubs and lost weight, only to put it back on and more when I stopped the diet. On this eating plan, you eat normally for five days then dramatically cut your calorie intake for two days.

I lost over a stone after the first two months, while my husband lost two stone over eight months. As it was a lifestyle change, not a diet, we've both kept the weight off after four years.

Doing it together has been great as we encourage each other when one of us wants to cheat, usually me! We walk around three miles each day, sometimes together, which gives us time to talk, too.

I've always liked sex but haven't always enjoyed it, experiencing years of thrush, bacterial vaginosis, frequent cystitis and urinary tract infections. These lead to vaginismus, when the vaginal muscles tighten, causing pain during penetrative sex. This happened because every time we had sex I'd think "am I going to be up all night on the toilet or itching the next day", causing me to tense up.

After researching this issue, I discovered that not using sexual lubricant was causing friction to my vaginal walls, leading to thrush. When we did use lube, the products we used contained glycerin (as do nearly all commercial lubes, and even some on prescription), which was exacerbating my thrush symptoms.

I also began to experience vaginal dryness in my early 40s, making me feel sore and uncomfortable. I now use organic lubricants, and all my symptoms have greatly decreased, transforming our sex life as it feels more comfortable and pleasurable. I can't imagine having sex without it!

However, several years ago I confess that my mind wasn't always focused when having sex and my husband would often say "where are you?"

It took a while for me to realise that I needed to switch the unwanted chatter off in my head and concentrate on what was happening to my body. It also seemed unfair to him as he has always been attentive to my sexual needs but got little back from me.

The lightbulb moment was when I decided to take charge in the bedroom, rather than lying on my back or waiting for him to initiate sex, much to my husband's delight.

Focusing on what is happening to my body and how his body makes me feel has led to me finding my G-spot at last and enjoying many blended orgasms, especially when I'm on top.

My lovely husband definitely noticed and thoroughly enjoys my sexual ministrations.

Losing weight together has boosted our sex life by making us both feel more body confident, leading us to explore new ideas, try sex toys and confide our sexual fantasies to each other, all of which has raised our sexual enjoyment. Even after all these years together we've been surprised to discover we share the same sexual fantasies but never told each other. I'm so pleased we have now!

I quite like the way I look now, something I probably wouldn't have said five years ago, and dress to suit my new shape rather than covering up with jeans and a baggy jumper.

Even if my libido decreases during the menopause I'm staying sex positive because I know there are many ways I can continue enjoying a great sex life whatever my age.'

Samantha Evans

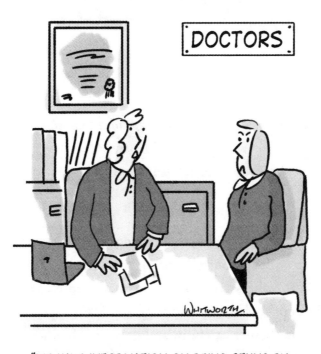

"WE HAVE INFORMATION ON BEING STUNG BY POISON DARTS, RARE TROPICAL DISEASES, AND CONTRACTING THE PLAGUE, BUT YOU CAN'T EXPECT US TO CARRY EVERYTHING ON THE MENOPAUSE."

8

Managing your menopause

'The menopause is the start of a new chapter
in your life. Enjoy it.'
Janet Rayment

Throughout this book, we've made reference to several ways you can help yourself during menopause. Some of these are medical, others are natural. In this chapter, we'll explore in more depth what your options are. We'd urge you to read through the chapter carefully, and do as much other research as you can before deciding on any particular path, whichever one is right for you.

You may believe in a firmly natural approach and decide you're going to avoid any type of medical intervention. And then discover that you're bleeding so heavily you will do anything, absolutely anything, to make it stop.

You may have always seen your GP and taken a pharmaceutical approach to your health but want to look at other options, or have decided that now would be a good time to make some adjustments to your lifestyle, too.

We have collated an overview of information from our team of experts. You don't have to pick one route and stick with it if it's not working. You don't have to pick any route. Or you could try a combination of whatever you think is best for you personally.

What we will say, and reiterate, is that if you're worried about any of your symptoms, please go and see your GP or menopause expert. Not everything is menopause-related when you're going through menopause, so it's best to err on the side of caution and get anything that's concerning you checked out.

THE MEDICAL APPROACH

HORMONE REPLACEMENT THERAPY (HRT)

It is important that you are fully aware of all the different treatment options available to you, including any potential benefits and risks, in order to make an informed choice. There are now many different treatments available, including different types of HRT that can be really effective at improving your symptoms and also your quality of life.

All types of HRT contain the oestrogen hormone. Taking HRT replaces the oestrogen that your ovaries no longer make after the menopause. Even low levels of HRT can have benefits in your body and improve your menopause symptoms.

There are different types of HRT and also different strengths, so the actual type of HRT can be tailor-made for each individual woman. It can be quite common for women to try two or even three types of HRT before they find one that suits them.

The prescribing of HRT has long been controversial. Over the past decade or so, some doctors have become reluctant to offer HRT and this has resulted in a lot of women not receiving HRT who would have really benefitted from it. In addition, many women have been unnecessarily worried about the perceived risks of HRT and so have avoided talking about their symptoms and asking their doctors for help.

However, in November 2015 the National Institute for Health and Care Excellence (NICE) guidelines on the menopause were published. So what do these NICE guidelines tell us? They provide clear statements regarding the benefits and risks of HRT. These have enabled healthcare professionals to be empowered with more knowledge and confidence to diagnose and manage the menopause.

Many women feel confused about the different types of HRT and also about the associated benefits and risks. HRT is actually much safer than most people realise, but it is important that your doctor takes your individual health into consideration when you're discussing HRT. Some women may choose not to take HRT and others may not be able to take it because of an underlying medical condition. If you are not sure whether or not you can take HRT, you should discuss this with your doctor, who may decide to refer you to a menopause expert.

NICE guidance states that HRT is the most effective treatment available to relieve menopausal symptoms such as hot flushes, night sweats, mood swings and bladder symptoms. For the vast majority of women starting HRT when they are under 60, the benefits outweigh the risks.

HRT is recommended for young women to take following an early menopause (see our chapter **What is 'premature' menopause?**) and they need to take it until they are at least 51. Otherwise, there is no set length of time for taking HRT. Some women take it for a few years to help improve their symptoms, while other women decide to take it for much longer. If your symptoms return when you stop taking HRT, this is not an effect of taking hormones, this is because you would still be having menopausal symptoms at that time if you had never taken HRT. The length of time you take HRT is usually an individual decision between you and your doctor.

Many women wait until their symptoms are really troublesome or even unbearable before starting HRT. However, taking HRT early really will make a difference to your symptoms and quality of life and also lead to a greater improvement in your heart and bone health.

HRT is not a contraceptive. If you still require contraception, you should talk to your doctor about the options available to you.

Types of HRT

HRT is available as tablets, skin patches or gel. The patches are usually changed twice a week and the gel is applied to your skin daily. The tablets are usually taken daily.

Except for those women who have had their womb removed, it is important that a progestogen (synthetic progesterone) is combined with the oestrogen. When you take oestrogen the lining of your womb can build up, which can increase your risk of cancer. However, taking a progestogen completely reverses this risk.

If you are still having regular periods, you will be given a type of HRT that means you continue to have a monthly period. This type of HRT needs to be taken for around a year. If you have not had a period for one year or have been taking this type of HRT for one year, it is likely you will be given a different type of HRT that means you will not have a monthly period. It can be common and completely normal to have some light bleeding or spotting in the first few months of using this type of HRT. However, if you experience heavy or prolonged vaginal bleeding, you need to inform your doctor.

If you have a history of a clot, migraine, diabetes or liver disease, you can still take HRT but it is likely that you will be recommended to use a patch or gel rather than a tablet. This is safer and associated with fewer risks compared to the tablet form of oestrogen. The progestogen is usually still given as a tablet, though, or in a Mirena coil.

There are many different preparations of HRT and even if one type doesn't suit you, for example if you experience side effects, it is very likely that another type will.

The oestrogen that is often prescribed is a type called 17 beta oestradiol. This is a 'body identical' oestrogen with the same molecular structure as the oestrogen that decreases in your body during the menopause. This type of oestrogen is available as tablets, in patches, gels and also in different types of vaginal preparations. It is also natural in that it is derived from a plant chemical extracted from yams, a tropical root vegetable.

Some older types of HRT contained a mixture of different types of oestrogens and were made from pregnant mares' urine. This type of HRT is 'natural' but it is not 'body identical' as it contains many types of oestrogens that we do not need in our bodies. This type of HRT is less often prescribed by doctors.

Micronised progesterone is a 'body identical' progestogen as it has the same molecular structure as the progesterone in our bodies. This means that it's usually associated with fewer side effects than other types of progestogens. Side effects of progestogens can include bloating, spots and mood swings. Micronised progesterone is also made from the yam.

Some 'natural' progesterone creams for your skin are available over the internet. These are not recommended as they are not absorbed into the body well and many do not contain enough of the hormone to be effective.

The risks of the hormones you are taking thus depend on the type of HRT and also your individual risk factors and health. It is very important that you are given the right type and strength of HRT for your individual needs and that the specific benefits and risks of your HRT are discussed with you by your GP or menopause doctor.

What are the benefits of HRT?

There are many benefits of taking HRT. Many women find that it gives them their lives back and once they have the right balance and strength of HRT, they are delighted. In addition, it can help to reduce the health risks associated with the menopause.

Many women find that all their symptoms improve within a few months of taking HRT. They often notice that their sleep improves, their mood improves and their concentration recovers. They also often notice that their energy is much greater than it was before they started taking HRT.

HRT usually works to stop hot flushes and night sweats within a few weeks. In addition, it will reverse many of the changes around your vagina and vulva, usually within one to three months, although it can take up to a year of treatment in some women. This means that HRT can improve symptoms of vaginal dryness and discomfort during sexual intercourse, help to reduce recurrent urine infections and also improve any increased frequency of passing urine. This is not a permanent change and without treatment then the symptoms usually return.

You may find that any aches or pains in your joints lessen and also that the texture of your hair and skin improves when taking HRT.

Your cardiovascular disease risk will reduce

HRT does not increase your risk of heart disease if it is started when you are under the age of 60. In addition, it does not affect your risk of dying from heart disease.

Numerous studies have shown that taking HRT, especially HRT with oestrogen alone, actually reduces the risk of developing cardiovascular disease (meaning heart attacks) in women. The benefits are greatest in those women who start HRT within ten years of their menopause. HRT can also lower your LDL cholesterol levels, which is beneficial for your heart and body.

Your risk of developing osteoporosis will reduce

NICE and International Menopause Society guidelines state that taking HRT can prevent and reverse bone loss, even for those women who only take low doses. This means that taking HRT reduces your risk of having a fracture due to osteoporosis. This benefit is maintained during treatment but does reduce when you stop taking HRT. However, there is some evidence that this reduction in risk of fracture persists for a length of time even when you stop taking HRT.

Other possible benefits

Some studies have shown a reduced risk of Alzheimer's disease and other types of dementia in women who take HRT. However, other studies have not shown this, so more work needs to be done in this area. In addition, some studies have also shown a reduction in the risk of bowel cancer in women who take HRT.

What are the risks with HRT?

Many women are scared of or worried about HRT because of the risks. There was a huge amount of media attention regarding the risks of taking HRT after the results of a large study about HRT, the Women's Health Initiative (WHI) study, were published over a decade ago. This study raised concerns over the safety of

HRT, particularly over a possible increased risk of breast cancer with HRT and also a possible increased risk of heart disease in older women who take HRT for the first time. However, the reporting of this study to the media was actually inaccurate and very misleading.

A recent study in 2016 suggested that the risk of breast cancer is slightly higher than previously thought; however, it appears that the type of progestogen is important, and the newer type of progestogen, micronised progesterone, was not mentioned in this study. It is so important for women to understand that there are many other risk factors for breast cancer. These include being overweight or obese, being older, drinking alcohol and smoking. A woman's risk of developing breast cancer when taking HRT containing an older type of progestogen is less than her risk of breast cancer if she drank two units of alcohol a night, was overweight or did not exercise. These lifestyle changes are all associated with an increased risk of breast cancer.

Your actual risk of developing the following diseases depends on many factors (such as your age, family history and general health), so not just whether or not you take HRT. This is why it is very important for your doctor to discuss the individual risks and benefits with you.

You can greatly reduce your risk of heart disease, stroke and many cancers by not smoking and by taking regular exercise and eating a healthy diet. These conditions become more common as you get older.

Breast cancer

This is the risk that most women worry about with HRT. You may have a small increased risk of breast cancer if you take HRT. However, if you are taking oestrogen-only HRT (so if you have had a hysterectomy), you are not likely to have an increased risk of breast cancer.

Taking combined (oestrogen and progestogen) HRT may be associated with a small increased risk of developing breast cancer. This risk increases the longer you have used HRT. The actual risk of breast cancer with taking combined HRT is very small, and less than the risk of breast cancer in women who are obese, who have never had children or who drink two to three units of alcohol each day. Studies into the link between HRT and breast cancer have not indicated any increased risk of dying from breast cancer in women taking HRT.

Any increased risk of breast cancer is reversed after you stop taking HRT.

Most of the studies carried out in this area have not shown an increased risk of breast cancer in women who take HRT for five years or less. Women who take combined HRT have an increased risk of having an abnormal mammogram, as HRT can increase the density of your breast tissue. This is not the same as increasing the risk of breast cancer.

It's important to note there is **no** increased risk of breast cancer in women who take HRT under the age of 51 as the woman is simply replacing the hormones their body should otherwise be producing.

Clots in the veins (venous thromboembolism)

A blood clot in the leg can cause a deep vein thrombosis (DVT). In some women, this clot may travel to your lung and cause a pulmonary embolism (PE). Together, DVT and PE are known as venous thromboembolism. Women who take HRT as tablets have a small increased risk of developing a clot compared to using oestrogen as a patch or gel. You are more likely to develop a clot if you have other risk factors for a clot. These include being obese, having had a clot in the past and being a smoker.

However, this risk of clot is not present if you use oestrogen as patches or a gel that is applied to the skin rather than tablets.

Stroke

NICE guidelines have shown that there is a small increased risk of stroke in women taking either oestrogen-only or combined HRT. However, there is no increased risk of stroke in women who use the patch or gel rather than tablets. In addition, oral HRT containing lower doses of oestrogen seems to be associated with a lower risk of stroke compared to those containing higher doses. Women under the age of 60 generally have a very low risk of stroke, whether they are taking HRT or not.

Are there any side effects of HRT?

Side effects with HRT are more likely to occur when you first start taking it and they usually settle with time. The most common side effects you may experience in the first few weeks are a feeling of sickness (nausea), some breast discomfort or leg cramps. These tend to go within a few months if you continue to use HRT.

Some women find that certain brands of HRT skin patches cause skin irritation. A change to a different brand or type of HRT may help. Various oestrogens and progestogens are used in the different brands. If you have a side effect with one brand, it may not occur with a different one. Changing the delivery method of HRT (for example, from a tablet to a patch) may also really help if you develop any side effects.

You should have regular follow-ups to decide whether you still benefit from taking HRT. If you are still experiencing menopausal symptoms on HRT, your dose will probably need to be increased.

Testosterone

Testosterone is another of the sex hormones that you produce. Many people think of it as the 'male' hormone, which is correct, but women need to have testosterone too. Testosterone is made in your ovaries and also your adrenal glands, which are small glands near your kidneys. Many women have low levels of testosterone as they go through the menopause.

Testosterone can be beneficial to improving your mood, energy, concentration and also sex drive (or libido). Low levels in your body are usually diagnosed by a blood test. Testosterone is usually given as a gel on your skin or sometimes as an implant. The dose of testosterone is very low so it will not cause facial hair growth. Testosterone is usually prescribed by a doctor who specialises in the menopause.

FACTS ABOUT HRT

You do not have to wait for your symptoms to be really bad or even unbearable before your doctor can give you HRT

Many women delay going to their doctor and asking for treatment as they feel that they are wasting their doctor's time and should wait until their symptoms are really bad. This is not the case, as HRT will help even if you have only mild symptoms. In addition, there is increasing evidence that the earlier HRT is started, the more you will gain protection from osteoporosis and heart disease.

HRT does not delay the menopause

Many women avoid taking HRT as they think they will then have their menopause later, after they come off HRT, but any menopausal symptoms you experience after stopping HRT are symptoms you would have experienced even if you had never taken HRT. So if you were going to have ten years of menopausal symptoms and took HRT for five years then you would still have five years of symptoms after stopping the HRT. Many women have menopausal symptoms for more than a decade and some women still have hot flushes when they are over 75 years old.

Some types of HRT are not associated with clots

If you take oral (tablet) HRT, there is a small increased risk of a clot developing in your leg or lungs. This increased risk is very small, this risk of clot is greater if you have other risk factors for developing a clot. These risk factors include being very overweight or having a history of a clot in the past.

However, if you take the oestrogen part of HRT as either a gel or a patch it gets absorbed directly into your body and is not then associated with an increased risk of clot.

Taking HRT can lower your future risk of heart attacks

Starting HRT when you are under 60 can actually lower your future risk of a heart attack. There is a very small increased risk of stroke in women who take combined HRT but this risk is reduced by using the oestrogen as gels or patches. The risk of stroke in women under 60 is usually very low, however, regardless of whether or not you take HRT.

You can take some types of HRT if you suffer with migraines

Many women notice that their migraines worsen as they go through their menopause due to changing levels of oestrogen. As you can't take the oral contraceptive pill if you have a history of migraines, many women (and doctors) incorrectly think that you cannot take HRT if you have migraines. If you have migraines, you should take oestrogen as gels or patches rather than as tablets. This is safe.

You do not have to stop HRT after five years

Many doctors encourage women to stop taking HRT after five years. However, there is actually no good scientific reason for this. Each woman needs to be assessed individually for the length of time they need to take HRT, depending on their risk factors and the benefits they are getting from HRT. The current guidelines are clear that there is no maximum age for taking HRT.

If you're under 51, you need to take HRT until you are at least 51, regardless of the age you are when you start taking it, as this is the average age of the menopause in women.

'Since taking HRT I am sleeping better and feel great. I have no more hot sweats.'
Tina

'I am amazed how much more energy I have. My joint pains have gone and I am enjoying life so much more.'
Kathryn

'My sexual relationship with my husband has returned. We are both delighted.'
Kate

BIOIDENTICAL HORMONE REPLACEMENT THERAPY (BHRT)

We are covering this because some women in the UK are now starting to use BHRT and there are also some forms available online so we think it's important to mention them.

Firstly, the NICE guidelines – the guidance your GP uses – state that the efficacy and safety of unregulated compounded bioidentical hormones (BHRT) are unknown.

In addition, the Advertising Standards Agency (ASA) issued a statement on 12 October 2017 about the way BHRT can and cannot be advertised.

Essentially there's a weight of scientific evidence that says HRT, including BHRT, is effective in treating symptoms of the menopause. Therefore straightforward adverts or statements that say they treat menopause symptoms are likely to be acceptable.

However, anyone offering BHRT will now need to avoid making claims that it is safer than HRT available through your GP. The ASA understands that there are no requirements for safety testing for HRT in compounded form e.g. BHRT, meaning that the relative safety is unknown.

In addition, the claim that BHRT is 'natural' is considered to be a problem. Although they are derived from natural products, they are still processed, e.g. in a compounding pharmacy.

Background to BHRT

In the 1940s, American chemist Russell Marker discovered he could replicate hormones using Mexican yams. Today, bioidentical hormones are based on a substance called diosgenin, which was originally derived from the Mexican yam but can also be derived from soya beans or synthesised in a laboratory.

Bioidentical hormones are plant based, although they may be mixed with non-vegan products during the compounding process. Bioidentical hormone medication is usually administered in the form of creams, lozenges, pessaries or capsules.

What is BHRT?

BHRT practitioners say that BHRT has an identical chemical and molecular structure to the hormones produced in the body so fits its hormone receptor sites ensuring that messages are translated properly and the effects are more consistent with the biochemistry of the body.

Bio-identical hormone prescriptions are personalised for every patient and it is important for a practitioner to initially assess a patient's medical history and symptoms. Tests include blood tests, pelvic ultrasounds, bone density scans and mammograms. They then prescribe a treatment plan and monitor a patient's progress, along with regular follow-up tests.

Where is BHRT available?

They are only available through private clinics and if you're considering using BHRT, check that the prescriber has the relevant medical qualifications.

There are now some forms of BHRT treatments available on the internet e.g. progesterone creams. If you're ordering from the internet there's the added risk that you don't always know the origin of the product or whether it's actually right for you.

Can I get BHRT on the NHS?

No. Some types of HRT are available on prescription from the NHS that have the same molecular structure as your body's hormones. Some doctors refer to these as 'body-identical', as 'bioidentical (BHRT)', which usually refers to compounded hormones, are not regulated and are not available to prescribe on the NHS.

We suggest you check with your GP first.

Knowing about your menstrual cycle is a good place to start. Whether you're having regular or erratic periods, or they've stopped altogether, it's wise to have an understanding of how your body works. Hormones aren't something to be afraid of, and the more you know the less you'll worry.

THE NATURAL APPROACH

If, for whatever reason, you don't want to take HRT and would rather manage your menopause entirely naturally, then you could take a look at your lifestyle – the suggestions below should help.

Your diet

If you've spent your life being able to eat what you want, when you want, without noticing any difference, you might find your perimenopausal years are a time of change. Many women notice some weight gain and find it harder to shift the pounds.

But your diet isn't just about keeping you in svelte shape. You can make some adjustments to what you eat and help to keep your hormones in balance. We're not talking faddy eating or quick-fix diets. This is about introducing changes – gradually if you like – to overhaul your eating habits once and for all.

We've already mentioned the stress hormone cortisol, and this, along with adrenaline, is produced by your adrenal gland. These two hormones are essential to your continued health and well-being, allowing you to respond appropriately to danger and external stresses such as family issues, relationships, work – essentially, life. But when these hormones are constantly raised due to 'life', they can play further havoc with the delicate dance of menopause hormones. One prime example is that the adrenal glands produce small amounts of oestrogen and progesterone as the ovaries decline, but they can't do this efficiently if in a constant state of high alert as the stress hormones have priority.

This in turn leads to internal stress – those symptoms we've discussed such as brain fog, fatigue and anxiety. So it makes sense to identify and manage your external stressors and reduce your internal stress – which is where good nutrition comes into play.

And if you're despairing reading this, thinking you'll have to spend your life eating lettuce, that's not the case at all. It's about replacing sugary, carb-laden food with delicious, filling and nutritious replacements. You can still enjoy treats, but women often find once they start on a healthier eating plan, they feel much less inclined to hit the biscuit tin.

Reduce your sugar and refined carb intake. Have you found that when you're under stress of any kind, when you feel out of control of your body, mind and life in general, you reach for the refined sugars and carbohydrates, alcohol, caffeine and processed foods? This is because your body is searching for something to make it feel good, get a quick fix, and these are easy, immediate solutions.

But have you also found that you can't just eat one biscuit or piece of chocolate? This is because the fix is short-lived, and you 'need' more to feel good again, raising both cortisol and adrenaline levels even higher. The more sugar you eat, the more insulin your body will produce – which in turn will send your hormones out of whack and make your menopausal symptoms worse. And the more sugar you eat, the more likely you are to be overweight, again a disruptor to your fine hormonal balance.

You might find it helpful to keep a food diary and note down your own triggers.

Stay hydrated. It's important to take in a minimum of two litres of water every day. Try a large glass with a slice of lemon on waking, another glass 20–30 minutes before food, and the rest throughout the day.

Nurture with nature. Eat a wide variety of foods of different colours found in nature, and include home-made juices and smoothies for a nutrient blast.

Introduce complex wholegrains, such as rolled oats, brown rice and quinoa.

If you have a sweet tooth, try indulging with mixed berries or melon instead of cake.

Try phytoestrogens, plant-based foods such as oats, barley, beans, lentils, yams, rice, alfalfa and mung beans.

Reduce your alcohol intake. Your liver metabolises waste oestrogen and ensures its production after the menopause, so it's important to keep it as cleansed as possible.

Eat more healthy proteins, such as nuts, eggs, fish, seeds, beans and lentils.

Stick to good fats, found in avocado, oily fish, coconut oil, nuts and seeds.

Supplement wisely. It's always wise to consult with a healthcare professional before taking any supplements or if you're on prescription medication. An important one to include is an omega-3 supplement, particularly if you don't consume foods containing these essential fats. Fish oils, krill oil, flax oil, there is something for everyone, often available in capsule or liquid form. And remember your daily recommended 10mcg of vitamin D.

Exercise

For perimenopausal women, the best type of exercise is high intensity interval training (HIIT), which usually involves 10–30 minutes of exercise – so is in shorter bursts than a traditional aerobics class. These should get you feeling hot, sweaty, out of breath and feeling the burn. Aim for three times a week. This type of exercise helps to slow or reverse the decline of your production of human growth hormone. Don't be put off by its name – you don't even need to go to the gym. Running up and down the stairs, doing some squats in the living room, skipping in the garden... it all counts. HIIT-style exercise reduces visceral body fat, boosts your immune system, improves insulin production, increases testosterone, improves bone density, increases muscle mass and reduces bad cholesterol.

You should combine this with lighter exercise, such as walking, two or three times a week. But really, when it comes to exercise, the best thing you can do is find what works for you and above all, something you enjoy.

If you'd like any more advice on nutrition or exercise, you should consider speaking to your GP or a specialist.

Complementary and herbal therapy

The NICE guidelines on the menopause state that doctors must explain to women that the quality, purity, constituents and results of these products may be unknown.

When choosing a supplement, it is a good idea to consult a nutritional therapist or herbalist. They will recommend food-state vitamins (those absorbed in the same way as when you're eating them in food), minerals and herbal supplements that are both safe and worth taking. Many supplements are not easily digested and you can end up spending a lot of money on products that basically end up in your urine or poo.

It's best not to buy supplements online unless you know the brands and they are manufactured in the European Union. If herbal supplements are made in the EU they must have a Traditional Herbal Remedies (THR) licence under Traditional Herbal Medicinal Products Directive (THMPD) regulations. This guarantees the manufacturer has acquired a licence that says they reach certain standards of manufacturing practice and that their products are tested to ensure they aren't adulterated. This is unlikely to change in the foreseeable future, regardless of changes within the EU.

For herbal products, a THR licence generally indicates quality of manufacture but doesn't necessarily guarantee that the product is right for you. In order to be sure that you have the right herbs for your health, you should consult a medical herbalist.

Products bought online from non-European sources are not supposed to be sold in the EU, but it's virtually impossible to police the ban. The reason non-European overseas supplements and herbal products are not allowed here is because a small but significant number have been shown to contain adulterants, incorrect species of plants and, in some cases, pharmaceutical drugs such as steroids or proton pump inhibitors (indigestion medicines).

See our **Resources** section to find a practitioner who can help.

Herbal treatments

We always recommend you contact a qualified medical herbalist and you can find one in your area through the National Institute of Medical Herbalists (see our **Resources** section) or you can check with them that a herbalist is listed as qualified. This is absolutely essential if you have a complex medical history, are undergoing treatment for cancer or have had cancer in the past, or are pregnant or considering becoming pregnant.

A herbalist's objective is to treat the body as a whole and each person as an individual. For this reason, it is difficult to give generic advice about how a menopausal symptom might be treated, as it will differ from woman to woman.

Herbalists use a combination of herbs that contain plant oestrogens, such as red clover and sage, and that affects the way the body produces oestrogen and progesterone, such as black cohosh.

The plant oestrogens (known as phytoestrogens) in sage and red clover may help to bolster levels of falling oestrodiol in your body, reducing symptoms of hot flushes, heavy bleeding and breast pain. There are two theories as to how this works. One is that they make the body think there is more oestrogen by binding to oestrogen receptors. The other is that by binding to oestrogen receptors, the phytoestrogens prevent oestrogens from being reabsorbed and increase the amount of circulating oestrogen.

There are many herbs that may help including:

Red clover (*Trifolium praetens*) is one of the most extensively studied food herbs and research indicates that it significantly reduces vasomotor symptoms (hot flushes) compared to a placebo. It is also thought to have psychological benefits.

Sage (*Salvia officinalis*) is used traditionally to reduce sweating at any age. Some women say that using a cold tea of sage helps to reduce menopausal night sweats. However, sage should not be taken in pregnancy because it helps to bring on and strengthen periods, so if you are trying to get pregnant during perimenopause it is best avoided.

Milk thistle (*Silybum marianum*) **and Blessed thistle** (*Cnicus benedictus*) are herbs that may help support the cells of the liver to work more effectively. This helps the gut to expel waste more easily. Milk thistle is safe to use alongside most medicines because it does not change the way that enzymes in the liver process drugs, and because it has no direct effect on the endocrine system it can be used in most cases of hormone imbalance.

Peony root (*Paeonia lactiflora*) acts on the balance between the pituitary gland, the hypothalamus and the ovaries and is thought to help balance the whole range of female hormones. It may be useful for uterine cramps as it reduces overactivity.

Tribulus (*Tribulus terrestris*) may help to increase testosterone in both men and women. Most testosterone in women is metabolised into oestrogen but women do need some testosterone to maintain strength, energy and vitality. Tribulus may have benefits in improving overall hormone balance and in particular in boosting energy.

St John's wort (*Hypericum perforatum*) is used primarily to help with nervous states such as depression and anxiety and some women say that it lifts their mood. As it increases the speed with which the liver clears out toxins, it is important not to use it alongside the oral contraceptive pill or other medicines such as antidepressants or immune-suppressing drugs because it may interfere with their effectiveness.

Black cohosh (*Actaea racemosa*) may reduce hot flushes and sweats in perimenopause and post menopause.

There were some concerns about the use of black cohosh after reports of liver failure in the United States. Careful assessment of the cases reported showed that the people who suffered were self-medicating. Some were buying pre-blended teas from unreliable sellers and others were picking and preparing their own. There was no accurate data as to how much was taken or for how long, and in each case there were other health problems and other doctor-prescribed drugs being taken. People treated by a qualified medical herbalist have reported no health problems.

If you have any history of liver disease, hepatitis or unstable liver enzyme tests, it is best to avoid this herb unless under the care of a qualified herbalist or doctor.

Red raspberry leaf (Rubus idaeus). Raspberry leaf is found in many gardens and you'll find it in most health food stores. You can safely pick leaves from raspberry bushes in your garden as long as they are away from family pet toilet areas. It may help improve the tone of the uterus and may relieve cramping and painful periods associated with menopause.

Hops (*Humulus lupus*). These may be useful to try in treating sleep disturbed by night sweats or hot flushes.

Marigold (*Calendula officinalis*). This herb is associated with wound healing and is also traditionally used to help improve circulation to the pelvic organs and is thought to improve uterine tone. Over time it may help reduce cramps and normalise menstrual bleeding. Marigold can also be used in the form of a pessary made with plant butters to help improve the health of the lining of the vagina, reducing dryness and increasing comfort during sex.

'I wish I'd known more about complementary health when I was going through the menopause. Herbs, minerals and vitamins can really help, plus rebalancing with traditional Chinese acupuncture along with massage and learning to take care of yourself. Women still seem to be the natural carers of the family but are hopeless about looking after themselves.'
Joanna Payne

'Why not try rocking the menopause with a daily exercise workout and diet with no sugar? It totally worked for me!'
Julia Annandale

WOMEN'S STORIES...

'Having had a total hysterectomy at the end of May 2016, I completely lost my mind! Seven weeks after the operation I was prescribed 150mcg of oestrogen, increasing this to 200mcg if I felt I needed to, and a blob of testosterone gel once a day. I was warned that this would not be a quick fix and that I may need to give it a few months to feel any real difference.

Thankfully this wasn't the case. Within about a week I had stopped crying and was already becoming more emotionally stable and felt more in control of my emotions. I started to sleep for longer periods at night and was able to make it through the night by about week three. Plus the hot flushes had nearly disappeared. I attended an appointment with my menopause doctor two weeks after starting the HRT and she could physically see the difference in me, commenting on how much brighter I seemed and how much more together I was.

I upped the oestrogen to 200mcg and things continued to improve. I could make normal decisions like what the evening meal was going to be. Sounds so silly now but I honestly became so frustrated and upset just by looking in the freezer trying to decide what to cook for my family. I got back on top of running my home and keeping up with the demands that having three children, a husband and two dogs bring!

I was in between jobs when I had my hysterectomy and went for various interviews post op but I turned them all down as I was convinced I wasn't capable or even worthy of accepting the position. I have since landed my perfect job and it's going really well, my confidence is returning with each passing day.

All of this is not to say I don't have bad days – of course I do – but I can tell if it's down to my menopause and I check all my medication is up to date. Normally I've forgotten to take my testosterone for a couple of days and that's generally the reason I've become weepy. Taking the HRT has taught me to be kinder to myself. HRT has given my children their mum back and my husband his wife back, but more than that it has given me *me* back.'

Rebecca Jones

WOMEN'S STORIES...

'The more I learn about the benefits of exercise during the perimenopause, the more committed I am to finding 30 minutes a day (or more when I have the chance!) for some sort of sport or exercise. I know how much happier I feel for it and I am starting to realise how it can help, physically, emotionally, mentally and socially.

I'm absolutely no super athlete, I'm unlikely to ever enter, never mind win a race, and my interest in sport has waxed and waned over the years. By the time I reached my late 40s, it was down to swimming on holiday and long walks with my sons at the weekend, when I could bribe them to join me.

Three years ago, when I was sleeping badly and feeling anxious and frazzled (both symptoms of perimenopause) a friend recommended indoor rowing. Within a couple of weeks I was sleeping through the night again and life seemed so much brighter.

I went on to row a million metres across 200 days and a marathon, 26.2 miles, five days before my 50th birthday, raising over £10,000 for Macmillan Cancer Support in memory of my mum.

Energised by this new lease of life, I founded a website dedicated to sharing stories of women in their 50s who love all sorts of sports, from ballet to cycling, yoga to powerlifting, endurance running to open water swimming.

I receive daily emails talking about the benefits of exercise for menopausal symptoms. From alleviating hot flushes (yoga is great apparently) to guarding against osteoporosis, something my mum had (it's important to include weight-bearing exercise such as running, lifting, walking or dance), experts agree exercise is hugely beneficial during and post the menopause.

For me personally, the greatest benefits focus on four things: sleep, mood enhancement and stress relief, achieving goals and making new friends.

Sleep. Many women going through the menopause talk about either finding it difficult to go to sleep or waking at 4am, their head full of worries. As an overthinker, this is a pattern I can easily fall into. Exercising, whether I'm swimming, indoor rowing, zipping around on my bike in the Dales or practising my yoga poses, helps me sleep. And a good night's sleep sets me up for the day ahead and all that I need to juggle as a mother, daughter, colleague, sister and friend. It's the bedrock of my energy and happiness.

Stress busting. The menopause hits us at a time in our lives when we are often the most pressed and stressed. Like many women, I'm part of the 'Sandwich Generation'. We are still caring for teenage children but also supporting ageing or unwell parents, alongside going out to work and looking after our homes. Sometimes this can be overwhelming.

On the days I carve out time, even in 15-minute bursts, for a brisk walk in the fresh air or on the rowing machine, my stress levels are always lowered and I simply feel more confident about my to-do list.

Achieving goals. In our 50s, as children leave home for university, careers or their own adventures, it's easy to feel a little lost and sense we are no longer needed as much as we were. Sport is a wonderful way to set new goals and revisit dreams we put on hold as our families grew. Many of the women who share their stories with me talk of finding themselves again having taken up a new exercise class, setting bigger challenges or even reinventing themselves with new careers as fitness instructors. A new sporting goal has a wonderful way of carrying us through the doubts and anxieties the menopause creates, physically and emotionally.

Making new friends. For me, one of the joys of sport is the women I meet and the chance to share, support and celebrate their dreams and achievements.

Sometimes this is done virtually through social media and sometimes I've been lucky enough to meet in person for a swim, bike ride or dinner. Some of the women I've met have set up their own women-only cycling or running groups. They are finding happiness in shared achievement (a 100km cycle, a new ballet performance) or simply going for a swim, walk or run together.

The menopause marks a physical change in who and where we are in our life's journey, and comes at a time when our social and family life changes. The friendship and community that sport gives us through this time is huge. We have people to talk to, dreams and worries to share, a sense that we aren't alone.'

Jo Moseley

9

What is 'premature' menopause?

'It hasn't (so far) been as bad as I thought it'd be… maybe I'm lucky. Still, it's difficult some days to accept that I'm at this stage of my life. I feel too young to be losing my vibrancy and "youth"… it doesn't seem fair when I feel I am now comfy being who I am… only to be changing in ways I don't want to.'
Karen Friend

The average age to go into menopause is 51, so if you're in your 40s, you're beginning to get prepared for the idea. But what if you're in your teens, 20s or 30s, the time when you're supposed to be in your fertile years? When you're thinking of starting a family and menopause should be far in the future?

There are two reasons for women to experience premature menopause. It can be as a result of surgery e.g. hysterectomy or oophorectomy, or illness e.g. as a result of chemotherapy, or it can happen naturally. Women under 40 years with early menopause are usually termed as having Premature Ovarian Insufficiency.

EARLY MENOPAUSE STORIES:

Jess was informed in her early 30s that she was in menopause just days after she'd been told she had ovarian cancer. It was picked up during her blood tests.

Debbie, at the age of 37, put her erratic and sometimes-missing periods down to having a high-powered job and the stress of a nasty divorce. She was told by the doctor that she was in menopause when she couldn't understand why she hadn't conceived with her new partner. She had to give him the news that 'staying with me could mean no children' (he did, and they're very happy).

Kate, again during investigations for fertility. Fortunately, she had one 'miracle egg', had her baby, and then crashed straight into the symptoms of menopause immediately after the birth. Try dealing with a newborn with menopausal symptoms going on too!

Cat, now in her early 30s, was diagnosed with POI at 15, and there is a debate whether she actually completed puberty, so is it menopause? Either way, she's been taking hormones for half of her life and is still 20 years younger than most women who go through menopause.

WHAT IS PREMATURE OVARIAN INSUFFICIENCY (POI)?

If you go through menopause when you're under 45, it is referred to as an early menopause. However, if you're under 40, it is referred to as Premature Ovarian Insufficiency (POI). Younger women who have gone through the menopause early have different health risks compared to older women and also have more benefits from taking HRT and other types of hormone treatment.

POI occurs when your ovaries no longer work properly when you are under the age of 40. Your ovaries no longer produce normal amounts of oestrogen and therefore may not produce eggs. This means that your periods either stop or become irregular and you may experience symptoms of the menopause.

However, in this condition, your ovaries do not usually completely fail and this is different to the menopause in older women. This means that the function of your ovaries can fluctuate over time, occasionally resulting in a period, ovulation or even pregnancy, sometimes several years after diagnosis. This intermittent or temporary return of ovarian function can result in around 5–10 per cent of women with POI being able to conceive.

Around one in a hundred women under the age of 40 in the UK have POI and it affects around one in a thousand women under 30. Many women have POI without realising and it is really important that if you have irregular periods or your periods have stopped, you should talk to your doctor about being tested and treated for POI.

WHAT CAUSES POI?

For most women with POI, the underlying cause is not known. However, the following will or may cause POI:

- Having your ovaries removed during an operation (known as oophorectomy).
- Having radiotherapy to your pelvic area as a treatment for cancer or receiving certain types of chemotherapy drugs that treat cancer.
- Having your womb (uterus) removed (a hysterectomy), even if your ovaries are not removed. Although your ovaries will still make some oestrogen after your hysterectomy, it is more common that your levels of oestrogen will fall at an earlier age than average.
- In around one in 20 women with POI, the condition is caused by an autoimmune disease. This means that your immune system (which normally protects your body from infections) mistakenly attacks itself. There may be people in your family who have other autoimmune conditions – for example, diabetes, thyroid conditions or Addison's disease.
- Some women with POI have genetic conditions. (Genetic means that the condition is passed on through families through special codes inside cells, called genes.) The most common of these is Turner syndrome, in which one of the female sex chromosomes (the X chromosome) is missing. Chromosomes are found in every cell in your body and contain genetic information. Genetic conditions causing POI are usually more common if there are other women in your family with POI or if you are under 20.

HOW IS POI DIAGNOSED?

The most common test for POI (and for early menopause) is a blood test to measure the level of FSH. If this is raised, it is very likely that you are menopausal. This blood test is repeated four to six weeks later. You may also be advised to have other blood tests – for example, some types of genetic tests. You may also be recommended to have a bone density test (DEXA scan) to determine the strength of your bones.

WHAT ARE THE SYMPTOMS OF POI?

The most common symptom for women with POI is that their periods stop. For around one in ten women, their periods do not even start and they present with POI at a very early age, usually under 20 years. Other women may notice that their periods become irregular. Many women with POI experience symptoms of the menopause. However, around one in four women do not have any of these symptoms.

It can be very common to feel anxious or even to have feelings of hopelessness after a diagnosis of POI has been made. Some women find they feel very sad and even guilty, as having POI can affect fertility.

Menopause symptoms can often have a very negative effect on your home and work life. It can be common for symptoms to come and go so you may have some months where you feel completely normal and then other times when you experience unpleasant symptoms that adversely affect the quality of your life.

WILL I NEED DIFFERENT TREATMENTS IF I HAVE POI?

Some women experience an early menopause due to premature ovarian insufficiency and this needs to be managed in a different way to 'normal' menopause.

What are the treatments available?

A healthy lifestyle is really important. Stopping smoking, eating a healthy, balanced diet and limiting alcohol can all be beneficial, as well as taking regular aerobic exercise. To reduce your risk of osteoporosis, eat a diet rich in calcium and do regular weight-bearing exercise. It is important to have adequate vitamin D levels to help keep your bones healthy. Vitamin D is made in the skin following sun exposure and is found in very small amounts in some foods. Many women need to take vitamin D tablets to maintain the correct levels in their bodies.

Many women find that they experience anxiety symptoms or even depression when they have an early menopause. You should not be ashamed if you have these symptoms. It is really important to talk about any symptoms you may be experiencing as there is effective treatment such as HRT available to help you.

All types of HRT contain an oestrogen hormone. Taking HRT replaces the oestrogen that your ovaries no longer make in the same quantities as when you were younger.

Without treatment in the form of hormones, there is a greater risk of conditions such as osteoporosis and heart attacks in younger menopausal women. It is very important if you are diagnosed with POI or early menopause that you receive hormones (HRT or the contraceptive pill) up to the natural age of menopause (51 years) to replace the hormones your body would otherwise be producing.

HRT is not a contraceptive. If you still require contraception, you should talk to your doctor about the options available to you.

There is no increased risk of breast cancer if you are taking HRT when you are young. Any risks that people may talk about regarding HRT are only relevant to those women who take it after the age of the natural menopause, which is around 51 years. So taking HRT when you are younger than 51 years gives your body all the benefits of HRT without the risks.

LONG-TERM HEALTH PROBLEMS THAT CAN ARISE FROM PREMATURE OR EARLY MENOPAUSE

Osteoporosis

Oestrogen helps to keep your bones strong and healthy. Your body has cells that build new bone and other cells that break down old bone. When there is less oestrogen in your body, bone breakdown occurs at a faster rate than bone build-up, resulting in a gradual loss of bone mass. Once this loss of bone reaches a certain point, osteoporosis develops. This leads to your bones becoming less dense and less strong.

People with osteoporosis have an increased risk of fractures occurring, even with little or no trauma. This can mean that normal stresses on your bones from sitting, standing, coughing or even hugging can result in painful fractures. These fractures can occur in any of your bones, including your spine, hips and wrists.

Cardiovascular disease

This means diseases of your heart and blood vessels, so includes heart attacks and strokes. Oestrogen is very important in keeping your blood vessels flexible and healthy as it seems to have a positive effect on the inner layer of the blood vessel walls. With the low levels of oestrogen in your body, your risk of cardiovascular disease increases.

Other changes in your cardiovascular system can also take place. Your blood pressure is more likely to start to increase. In addition, bad cholesterol, or LDL cholesterol, levels may increase and good cholesterol, or HDL cholesterol, may decline.

POI needs managing in a different way to a regular menopause. You'll find more information about treatment options in the **Managing your menopause** chapter.

THE DAISY NETWORK

The Daisy Network was created in 1995 to provide support to women who have been diagnosed with POI, along with their families and partners.

They understand that this diagnosis can feel incredibly isolating and often women are left confused and unsure where to go next.

This charity provides information and the latest research findings on various aspects of POI including HRT and other treatment options, managing the longer-term health implications such as bone and cardiovascular health, nutrition, and the psychological impact. And it also helps women find out more about egg donation, adoption or how to lead a childless life positively.

You'll find their details in our **Resources** section.

SURGICAL MENOPAUSE

Although most women go through menopause naturally, many women have their menopause early as the result of an operation. The operation in which both ovaries are removed causes an immediate menopause. The onset of your menopause is very sudden and abrupt compared to the natural menopause. Recovering from an operation can take time and then experiencing

that your body would otherwise be producing. HRT is the most effective treatment to relieve symptoms caused by the menopause such as hot flushes, night sweats, mood swings and bladder symptoms.

Many women are under the age of 51 when they have surgery to remove their ovaries. When you have your ovaries removed under the age of 45, your body's requirements for hormones is greater compared to older women. This means that you typically require much higher doses of these hormones (typically oestrogen) than if you are older, so if you are given HRT and are still experiencing menopausal symptoms after your operation, the most likely reason is that your HRT dose is too low. Many young women actually need two or even three times more HRT than the average dose given to older women.

Your doctor or menopause expert may recommend that you have blood tests after your operation to determine the levels of hormones in your body. This can be useful for some women who are experiencing menopause symptoms. There are different types of HRT and different ways to administer it e.g. tablet, patch or gel. Some women do not absorb some types of HRT well, so if your levels of oestradiol (a type of oestrogen, see page 24) are low despite you receiving a high dose of HRT, it is likely that your doctor will recommend changing the type of HRT you're on until you find the one that works best for you.

Testosterone is also a very important hormone for women. This hormone is made in your ovaries and also your adrenal glands, which are small glands near your kidneys. This means that after your operation testosterone will only be made in the adrenal glands, so you will experience a reduction in the amount of testosterone in your body.

As a result, you may find that your mood, energy, concentration and also sex drive are negatively affected. Although taking oestrogen can help, it is often taking testosterone that really improves these symptoms. Many women notice that their mind is clearer and more focused when they take testosterone.

Testosterone is usually given as a gel, which you rub into your skin, usually on your lower abdomen or thigh. It can also be given as an implant. It can sometimes take a few months for the full effects of testosterone to work in your body.

'I had breast cancer at 36 and had to take the tamoxifen drug. This put me straight into an early menopause with no warning at all. I only had my consultant to talk to at that stage. In the end the symptoms lasted about five years and I still get mild hot flushes 18 years later.'
Anonymous

WOMEN'S STORIES...

'At the age of 41 I was plunged headfirst into a brutal, burning menopause.

I'd just finished five months of surgery for breast cancer and starting on hormone therapy seemed like a breeze by comparison. Back then, I used to think myself "lucky to be alive" and feel grateful that my life had been preserved by the NHS.

Looking back, I see that luck had nothing to do with it. I'm entitled – just like everyone else – to a happy healthy life and although I do remain forever grateful for the care I received, it's got nothing to do with luck.

For two years after my surgery, I went to my GP once a month for a jab into my tummy. It hurt, a lot. The injection was part of my treatment, which lasted for five years in all. There was very little information, support, or advice, other than being advised to avoid all plant-based remedies that contained oestrogen, because my particular strain of breast cancer was hormone receptive. Oestrogen was my enemy and my treatment was to banish it from my body. The result was that I was plunged into surgical menopause.

Embracing my new, post-menopausal world, I acquired a series of layered clothing which I could variously peel on and off when the glow kicked in. I've heard it called Tamoxifen Glow, but for me it was more like a steel furnace burning in my chest which radiated out like molten lead in just a few seconds.

I couldn't sleep, I played the hokey-cokey with my duvet, left arm in, right leg out and shake the whole thing about. Having quit my job, I went back to university to study horticulture and dodged between freezing cold greenhouses and hot classrooms. Boiler on/boiler off. Jumper on/jumper off.

I felt embarrassed. What an understatement. I was mortified, feeling isolated that I couldn't tell anyone what was really happening to me. I hadn't yet discovered the benefits of a menopause wing woman who could see me turning a beetroot colour and show me some love. I even joked, "If I'm lucky, I'll get to do the menopause twice," meaning that if I was well enough to make it into my 50s, I might be able to have a natural menopause.

I almost made it, the natural part that is. I was distinctly in perimenopause age 50 when I had a recurrence of breast cancer. Same side, same treatment more or less, just the older lady version. So off I went into menopause land again. Whereas the first time it was just another life hurdle to jump, this time it made me grumpy. I mean, really grumpy, because this time I knew there was no coming back. Fertility, kaput, gone.

Worse still, given all the other things I've overcome with my health, it still never makes it to the top of the pile, I just put up with it, because I have to. I also rationalise that I would've been in natural menopause anyway, but I'm grumpy because I didn't have a choice. I take Starflower oil and a calcium tablet each day, because old lady cancer treatment rots your bones, and by and large I just get on with it.

In April 2017 I attended the Nottingham Breast Institute to review my treatment, which I'm delighted to say came to a conclusion. I've been discharged after a total of 15 years attending the clinic each year. It means no more tablets, and for the first time, entering the normal health population for breast cancer screening. It's been a long haul, and life feels very different now, mostly for the better. I'll never know how a natural menopause would have impacted on me. Instead I'm focusing on being out on the other side of it, and accept it as one of the necessary impacts of protecting my health and well-being for the future.'

Sue Pringle

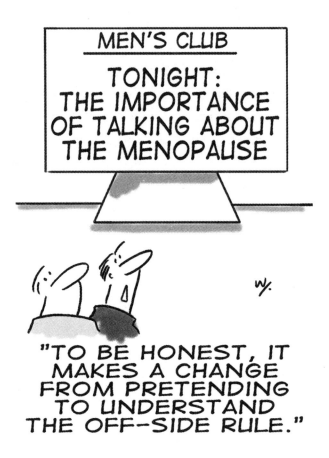

10

Maintaining healthy relationships

'It's about time people started talking about menopause more. My wife was climbing the walls with it, won't talk about it and I haven't got a clue what to do.'
Anonymous London taxi driver

Healthy relationships play a big part in our happiness. And if menopause brings challenges, our relationships can sometimes be a casualty. This isn't just with a 'significant other' – although these close relationships are often the ones most obviously affected. But our relationships with children, parents, wider family, friends and colleagues can sometimes feel the effects, too.

If menopausal symptoms are causing you to suffer, support from your network of family, friends, colleagues and manager is vital. Which means keeping the lines of communication open, being as honest as you can with those around you and leaning on your nearest and dearest if things become difficult.

During your life there will have been people you have supported over the years, and the chances are they'll be more than happy to help you when it's your turn to ask for support. Remember, if you don't tell anyone how you're feeling through the menopause and why, they can't read your mind – talking about it really does help. In particular, your partner and your children, if you have any (and depending on their ages), will know that there's something amiss and will want to help, but they won't necessarily know how. It really is a good thing to talk to them openly, involve them wherever possible and help them to understand. As menopause still isn't talked about openly, there can be a lot of unnecessary worry – it's time to demystify menopause and make it a normal topic of conversation. Let people help you as you would help them. You'll find it serves to make your relationships stronger.

In this chapter, we explore how relationships can be affected by menopause and how you can make sure these relationships not only stay healthy but can even be improved as you journey through menopause and beyond.

HOW DO I TALK TO MY PARTNER ABOUT MENOPAUSE?

We've mentioned the importance of communication and discussion, but it can sometimes be difficult to know how and when to do this. Menopause is a time when patience can be tested and understanding is needed. It's useful for partners to recognise that any mood swings, distress and anxiety are not really anything to do with them. Sometimes, though, this is easier said than done. Being there emotionally is a skill that requires individuals to suspend their own emotional needs, not to try and 'fix it' but to simply be there. It's more than empathy.

You might find it easy to talk to your partner about anything and having a discussion about menopause won't be a problem for either of you. For others, though, it can be a little more tricky and it's worth putting in some prep to get the best out of the chat.

Remember, your partner may not know much about menopause. Before you try to talk to them about it, perhaps you could share this book with them, or talk to them about what you've learned.

Here are some tips for starting the conversation. You might not need to use all of them, but they can be helpful in getting you started:

- **Find the right place**. What's best for you? Sometimes it can feel easier to have a conversation in a public place, like a café or restaurant. Or you might prefer the privacy of your home.
- **Choose the right time**. Some people like to talk at the end of the day, while others feel too tired by then. Consider what's best for you both.
- **Prepare the ground.** Tell your partner you want to talk about menopause, so you are both focused on the discussion when the time comes.
- **Think carefully about what you want to say.** It can be useful to write things down.
- **What do you want from your partner?** Communication is a two-way process, so you need to consider what their response might be.

Communication isn't always easy, even with those we love and share our lives with. While we might easily have conversations about day-to-day life, talking about more personal or intimate matters can be more difficult. But it's vital to be heard, and to listen.

Try these tips to improve your communication skills:

- **Use 'I' statements** e.g. 'I feel self-conscious about my body at the moment and it will really help me if you're sensitive to this.' You can then discuss together how you can address the way you feel.
- **Take turns to talk and to listen.** If the conversation starts to become difficult, remember it's important to listen as well as to be heard. You could set a time limit for each of you to talk and the other to listen.
- **Paraphrase what you are both saying.** After one person has finished talking, the other could try paraphrasing what they've just heard – 'So to me it seems like you are saying…' This way you know that your partner is taking in what you're saying and understanding what you're asking of them, and in turn you can talk through any issues or questions they may have.
- **Practise.** Communication is a skill to be learned like any other. By building positive habits into your conversations with your partner, you will find it increasingly easier to make yourself heard, and in turn for your partner to give you the support you need during menopause.

MY MOOD SWINGS ARE REALLY IMPACTING MY RELATIONSHIP, WHAT CAN I DO?

If you're suffering from mood swings, it can be difficult for those around you to cope with the changes. Remember, you are still you and these mood swings won't last forever. But how to manage when they strike?

- **Name the mood swings.** As in, tell your partner that you're biting their head off because you're in an irritable mood. 'It's not you, it's the menopause' can actually help them cope more constructively than if they think you're not telling them something.
- **Try time out.** If you're feeling angry or irritable, it could be a good idea to take some time out, just be by yourself in a different room to your partner for a while and give yourself some space to relax.

Communication and discussion under the guidance of a relationship therapist can help you to work things through together. See our **Resources** section for information on finding a therapist.

WHY HAVE I STARTED TO FEEL SELF-CONSCIOUS ABOUT MY BODY?

Sometimes, menopause can make us feel concerned about our bodies, with insecurity and self-consciousness striking where we may previously have felt confident. 'I went through an early menopause and felt like I'd turned into an old hag overnight' is a common phrase we hear. Feeling awkward or anxious about your body can sometimes lead to avoiding sex.

But try to remember that your partner is making love to all of you – if you have been together for a long time, attraction is not just about looks, but about your shared experiences and the life you've created together.

If you have become self-conscious when you never were before, your partner may find this hard to deal with. This is where you need to communicate openly, as blanket reassurance from them is not usually helpful – it's often not enough for them to offer platitudes like 'you always look lovely'. Often a practical approach can help. For example, ask them to be sensitive to what would make you feel less self-conscious – perhaps making love with the lights off, or partially clothed. Patience and understanding is much more effective than irritation in helping one another to relax and forget body concerns. Remember, body shape alters with age and it's important not to put undue pressure on yourself with unrealistic expectations. Being able to share your thoughts with a non-judgemental, supportive partner really helps.

Your partner is your equal, and as you journey through life together you will each bring challenges to the relationship that you need to address together. As with any other life change, the menopause is something to approach together, examining the effects on you both and working on the best ways to handle and overcome any hurdles.

WHAT IF SAME-SEX PARTNERS ARE GOING THROUGH MENOPAUSE AT THE SAME TIME?

The important thing to remember for partners is that even though they may both be going through menopause; they may not be experiencing it in the same way. One may have hot flushes and night sweats. The other may have irritability and anxiety.

The key as ever is communication and understanding. It's important to remember that this is a transitional period and you will get through it. Women going through the menopause together can have a positive effect on one another, having a partner who can identify and sympathise with the symptoms and feelings through first-hand experience.

WILL I LOSE MY SEX DRIVE?

We have explored this more fully in the chapter, **What will happen to my sex drive?** But it's hard to write a chapter on relationships without also talking about sex. The changes in your hormonal balance can sometimes lead to loss of libido, and if you're suffering from a lack of body confidence too then it can be difficult to feel as if you're sexually attractive. But the idea that the menopause signals the end of a woman's sexually active years is fast losing ground. Sex is no longer a purely procreational activity. As most women can expect around a third of their life to be post menopause, it's important to realise that a healthy, satisfying sex life can still exist once you've gone through the menopause. For some women, menopause brings a sense of sexual liberation.

And even if your sex drive does dwindle a little, that's not necessarily bad news, as one woman told us: 'I've always had a higher sex drive than my partner, but as I've aged I have found my need for sex to be less. I don't fancy my partner any less, but now it feels as if we are at the same place regarding desire and frequency of sex.'

For some women, the declining levels of oestrogen result in less vaginal lubrication, which can result in intercourse becoming painful (dyspareunia), and in anticipation of pain may also cause some women to develop vaginismus (a reflex where the muscles of the vagina contract such that penetration isn't possible). See our chapter on **What is vaginal dryness and urinary incontinence?** for more on this.

These conditions can cause a woman to want sex less, coupled with a low appreciation of her body image, or the perception that her partner is less interested. Partners can then feel rejected and this can cause them to give up initiating sex, creating a physical distance between the couple.

For many couples, going to bed together at the end of the day is a time to catch up, chat and cuddle, and is often the only time they have to be close and physical. If night sweats or insomnia are getting in the way, some couples choose to sleep apart. While this might feel like a good practical solution, it can create further physical distance and make couples feel isolated from each other if there isn't any other physical intimacy in their relationship.

If you find that your usual sexual activity isn't working for you any more, you could talk to your partner about experimenting with different sexual positions that would make intercourse more comfortable.

MASKING OTHER PROBLEMS

The menopause can mask other sexual problems. For example, if a man is experiencing difficulty with his erections he may have withdrawn from sexual contact and could feel relieved that his partner wants less sex than before.

Biological problems often account for sexual problems in menopausal women. It is important to recognise that these problems hardly ever exist in isolation. Psychological, sociocultural, and/or relationship issues may also contribute to difficulties experienced by women and therefore it's important that a thorough assessment is made to address these and other non-physiological factors.

See our **Resources** section for information on finding a therapist.

SHOULD I TALK TO MY CHILDREN ABOUT MENOPAUSE?

If you have children living with you, the chances are they'll have noticed if you are suffering from menopausal symptoms. Talking to them about menopause, if they are old enough to understand, can reassure them that you are going through a perfectly normal process. Remember, though, your children may not want to acknowledge your sexuality, or may feel uncomfortable with the notion of you getting older, so it's important to be sensitive in your conversations with them. However, children can prove a source of support, to both you and your partner.

OTHER IMPORTANT RELATIONSHIPS

If you can, you might find it helpful to talk to your own mother about her experience of menopause, as the age she reached menopause could influence your own journey. She could also give you valuable advice on how she coped, or simply just provide a listening ear. Your symptoms and how you manage them may not be the same, but it's good to share the experience.

Friends are also invaluable. You might go through menopause together, or at completely different times, but having support and camaraderie from your friends can often lift your spirits.

MANAGING LIFE CHANGES

Navigating your relationships as you journey through menopause can sometimes be rocky. There may be lots of other changes occurring in your life at this time. We talk about the 'sandwich generation', those who are looking after elderly relatives at the same time as supporting children making their way in the world. And there are other life experiences, such as changing jobs, moving house, experiencing bereavement or relationships breaking up. Understandably, these can all add extra stress in your life and may hit at a time when you're feeling less able to cope. It can be difficult to know whether what you're feeling is down to these events, the menopause, or both.

WHAT DO MEN THINK ABOUT MENOPAUSE?

Menopause isn't a 'women's issue' to be kept within the confines of the sisterhood. As we've explored in this chapter, talking openly about the menopause to the men in your life – partner, husband, father, son, friends, work colleagues and managers – is the best way to explain just how you're feeling, and why.

To understand more about men's perceptions of menopause, we asked 100 men for their thoughts. And some of the fears that women tend to have are just that: fears, not reality. Asked whether menopause makes a woman less attractive or sexy, the response was a resounding 'no', with one respondent saying 'just as appealing' and another saying 'more!'

When it came to understanding the menopause, all of our respondents knew what it was, and many had an idea of some of the symptoms, with one saying 'it's a nightmare for some' and another realising there is 'no universal effect as everyone is different and will respond differently'.

And while women often worry that men view menopausal women in a certain light, it seems that this isn't really the case, with many of our respondents saying they had no 'perceptions' or 'preconceived ideas' and one interestingly commenting that 'I never perceive it as a positive thing as it isn't portrayed this way by females.'

In terms of supporting their partner, most men are keen and willing to help, with answers to 'Would you know how to help a woman going through menopause?' ranging from 'Not particularly but I would be willing to learn' and 'Mainly love, reassurance and understanding' to 'Openness in a relationship should mean you can talk about anything. Men have age-related issues too!'

So it seems that, in some cases, many of the perceptions of menopause may stem from our own insecurities and fears. Let's take heart in this quote from one of our respondents: 'I love my partner so much that the menopause won't change this.'

WOMEN'S STORIES...

'Late in 2015, I could never have imagined that my life was about to change beyond all recognition. Paul – not his real name – came for a meeting, and after 12 years on my own, I knew I'd just met the most wonderful man. There was nothing to judge, only appreciate.

We started to develop a lovely friendship. It was so easy. That was the most amazing thing. I didn't feel the need to impress him or to try and figure out how I should act to get him to like me.

But then, confusingly, I felt vulnerable like I never felt before.

I started to over-analyse what he said, what I said, what I was thinking, what I thought he thought. As his messages became more romantic, I became more insecure.

My limiting beliefs about my attractiveness began to overwhelm me. Suddenly I was wondering about my body. It had been ages since I last wondered about my body.

I have scoliosis so it looks a bit off-centre – that, plus the changes inevitably brought about by age – well, I was 71. The good news is, I look really good dressed. I didn't think anyone was going to see me naked.

But I was beginning to feel distracted all the time. Even more unsettling, I was experiencing sexual feelings again. I hadn't been with a man in nearly 20 years so I was starting to worry that it was too late – you know what they say, "if you don't use it, you lose it."

I truly believed I had everything I wanted, including the love of my friends. There was nothing missing. But on that day, I felt like I was whole even though I believed I already was.

I knew I wanted to be with him – I can't remember ever really wanting to be with a man. I was 71 and I hadn't had sex in 20 years.

All the insecurities came back – about my body, about having sex, about not being good enough in bed. Just in case, I thought it might be a good idea to buy one of those vaginal lubricants.

In the end, I was the one who crossed that line. "I want you to come to bed with me," I told him. And we did.

All my fears flew out of the window. There was so much love, so much gentleness, so much care, so much patience. As it turns out, I didn't need any lubricants. He thought my body was beautiful – I thought he was either mad or blind but I decided to believe him. That's probably one of the greatest gifts I gave myself – and him. To believe him.

We've been together eight and a half months. I trust him as I never trusted another man. I feel totally accepted. I feel totally safe. I never felt like that before. I can't believe it!

We both have very similar life experiences, moving on from unhappy marriages to creating a good life for ourselves.

We both have a need to use our knowledge, skills, experience and gifts to help others. It gives us both a feeling of accomplishment and purpose.

We both have very similar needs and wants. But we're not clones of each other either.

We're different enough to enjoy really interesting conversations, to be open to each other's point of view. Neither one of us have the need to defend our position to the death nor to be right at all costs.

I like him just the way he is and I, too, feel totally accepted – and appreciated. It's an awesome experience.

There's a lot of truth in the saying, "Start as you mean to go on." I really believe that you can only do that if you know and like yourself. That's how you can trust yourself to make choices that really work for you. That's how you know that you're worthy of true love, that you deserve to be accepted.

You know you're in the right place when you're not made to feel you'd be okay if you'd only tweak a little bit of this and a little bit of that.

And the same is true for this other person, the one you say you love.'

Sue Plumtree

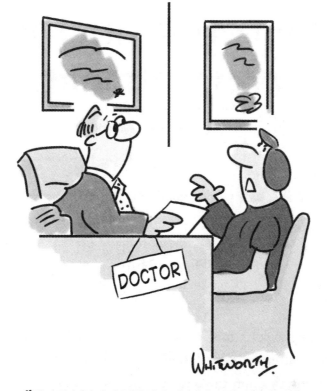

"I KNOW HOW LONG IT TAKES
TO GET AN APPOINTMENT, SO
WE'LL BOTH SIT HERE UNTIL
MY MENOPAUSE STARTS."

11

Getting the best from your doctor's appointment

'Menopause? Why not call it "womenopause?"
Time to stop, take stock and then "womenostart"
the next exciting stage of life!'
Denise Hunt

Talking to your doctor about the menopause can sometimes feel intimidating. With GP appointments at a premium, just getting through the door can feel like a battle these days. And when the doctor asks you what's wrong before the door has even closed, it can be daunting to say the least to launch into the reasons you're there.

In May 2016, a survey conducted on behalf of the British Menopause Society (BMS), has revealed that one in two women in Great Britain, aged 45-65 who have experienced the menopause in the past 10 years, had not consulted a heathcare professional about their menopause symptoms. This is despite women surveyed reporting on average seven different symptoms and 42% saying their symptoms were worse or much worse than expected.

But your GP should be there to help. In this chapter, we'll examine what is within a GP's prescribing power and explain the guidelines they are working within. You need to prepare to get the best from your valuable GP appointment, so here are a few pointers on the type of things you could be asking. Most appointments are fairly short, but we can help you get the most out of every minute by figuring out what to say so you can walk out with answers to your questions.

WHAT ARE THE NICE GUIDELINES?

The National Institute for Health and Care Excellence (NICE) is a non-departmental public body that develops guidelines for health and social care based on evidence. Accountable to the Department of Health, NICE is nevertheless an independent organisation.

It's important to note that the legislation surrounding NICE means its guidance is only officially for England. The organisation does have agreements in Wales, Scotland and Northern Ireland, with devolved administrations making the decisions on how to use the guidance.

Under the guidelines, your medical practitioner should involve you in decision-making and give you enough information to help you make your own choices.

These guidelines will be used by your GP or other healthcare professional to determine how they speak to you, assess you, make necessary diagnoses and what type of medical treatments and interventions they are able to offer you.

This includes:

- Talking to you about lifestyle changes, how to manage your symptoms and the long-term implications of menopause.
- Offering advice on HRT, non-hormonal treatments such as clonidine (which can help with hot flushes) and non-pharmaceutical methods such as Cognitive Behavioural Therapy (CBT).
- Giving you information about contraception throughout perimenopause and postmenopause.
- If you are likely to go through menopause due to medical or surgical treatment, informing you about menopause and fertility before your treatment and referring you to a specialist.
- Suggesting testosterone supplements if you have experienced a severe drop in sex drive, and localised vaginal oestrogen if you are suffering from vaginal dryness.
- Explaining that while you may wish to use complementary therapies and treatments, the safety of these cannot always be guaranteed.
- Pointing out that the efficacy and safety of unregulated compounded bioidentical hormones (BHRT) are unknown.
- Talking to you about the importance of regular health, breast and cervical screening.
- Giving you more information on the types of medication you can take if you have breast cancer, diabetes or are in a high-risk category for clotting conditions and thrombosis.
- Offering advice on bone health and osteoporosis.

This is a small snapshot of the guidelines. We've included links to the full set of guidelines in the **Resources** section.

I'M WORRIED MY DOCTOR WON'T TAKE ME SERIOUSLY. HOW CAN I GET THEM TO LISTEN TO ME?

We all know that getting in to see your GP can be a fairly difficult task, with clinics offering urgent appointments, telephone-only appointments and call-back systems. For some, a general appointment might not be available for several weeks.

But it's important not to let red tape stop you from going to see your GP.

GPs have to be able to deal with a huge variety of different issues and it's a fact that they simply can't all be good at all of them. Women's health is a hugely challenging area and you don't need specialist gynaecological training to be a GP. So your doctor's knowledge will vary, depending on the level of training they've had in this area.

However, that's not to say there's nothing you can do. If you feel your doctor is unhelpful you can request to see another doctor at your practice, who will not necessarily share the same views. Now is also a good time to make friends with the receptionists at your practice. Ask them who the best person is to speak to about menopause. It might be a different GP to the one you usually see, or it could be a nurse practitioner.

It comes down to which doctor has had the most training in menopause, and for that matter who is most interested in it. It will be a hugely individual thing across the nation and across different regions and practices, so do your homework, ask around and book in an appointment to see who is considered to be the best person to talk to about menopause.

I ONLY GET TEN MINUTES WITH THE DOCTOR IF I'M LUCKY. HOW CAN I SAY EVERYTHING I NEED TO?

There is great pressure on GP surgeries, which can put non-urgent appointments further down the list – this is why you'll sometimes find it hard to get an appointment very quickly. Currently, GP appointments are about ten minutes long. And when you want to talk about hot flushes, mood swings, vaginal dryness and heavy bleeding, it might not feel like long enough – let's be honest, it can be very difficult to get the words out when you're talking about intimate matters.

But your GP is a professional and has heard it all before. To get the right treatment you need to describe your symptoms, so please don't be afraid to talk about what's bothering you. Armed with the right information, you can use your appointment time very wisely. You've seen in this guide some of the treatment options available, so you can say to your doctor you'd like to try HRT, or you have heard that localised vaginal oestrogen can help with dryness, for example, or that you'd like a Mirena coil fitted to stem your heavy bleeding. Read and learn as much as you possibly can in advance, so you can confidently talk to your doctor or nurse about what you'd like from them. Always ask for your GP's opinion. They know your medical history and can explain your options and any associated risks.

Some surgeries offer longer appointments if you think you need them, so if you really feel your usual appointment length won't be enough, ask the receptionist to book you in for back-to-back appointments if they are available. If you think you'll still struggle, set a plan and prioritise your symptoms rather than tackling them all at once.

Ultimately, if you think your GP isn't taking you seriously then go and see someone who will – it could be another doctor in the same surgery. Don't give up and never feel that all options have been closed to you.

IS THERE SUCH A THING AS A MENOPAUSE CLINIC?

It depends where you live. Unfortunately, NHS funding means these aren't available everywhere. There are some available, and it's worth checking to find out if there's one near you – it might not be in your immediate vicinity, but you could be able to get a referral to your nearest one.

If you feel you need extra, specialist support that isn't available to you on the NHS, it may be something you need to consider paying for.

'I feel like my old self again. I can concentrate and multitask again. It is fabulous. I know there are some risks of HRT for some women but for me the benefits are huge.'
Louise

WOMEN'S STORIES...

'My body was changing before I even realised it was happening. The first thing I noticed was my skin. I have cleansed and moisturised my face and neck morning and evening since my early 20s. Suddenly the cream was being taken in to my skin on contact. I thought the manufacturers must have changed the product, but no, they hadn't.

It isn't an exaggeration to say I was using three times more. The colour of my normally very pale white skin changed. I would never hold a tan before, now I have to protect my skin from direct sunlight. The positive change is no more periods.

I have never been offered HRT. In fact, neither doctor I saw over the time period of going through the change ever talked to me about menopause.'

Jane Taylor

'Menopause is not the end or even the beginning of the end. The menopause is when a woman becomes the wise crone of the community in the nicest possible way, and this should be celebrated more.'
Linda Booth

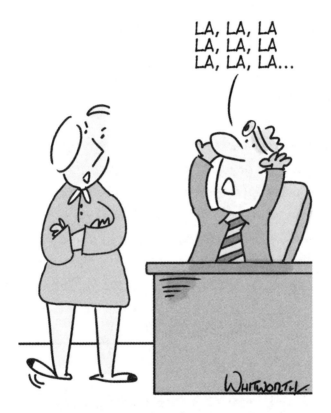

"I'M BEGINNING TO THINK
YOU'RE NOT LISTENING TO ME."

12

Menopause and work

'I am in no doubt of the benefits to my officers and staff, and to the public policing serves, of a menopause in the workplace policy and practice. It has resulted in reduced absence and staff turnover, together with providing vital information to men and women in my organisation. Quite simply it is the right thing to do. In doing so we have broken the last taboo.'
Sue Fish, former Chief Constable of Nottinghamshire Police

More and more of us are working until later in life. We're working for longer, the state retirement age has increased and you can work for as long as you like. We not only have longer careers, but more women are in senior positions and either need to work for financial reasons or simply want to work. In fact, 75–80 per cent of women of menopausal age are at work.

Around one in three of the workforce in the UK is over 50. So not only is it important for employers to retain the valuable investment they've made in their employees, it's also important we can perform at our best and enjoy our work life. According to a survey in 2016, one in four women had considered leaving work because they couldn't cope with their menopause symptoms. For an employer that would mean losing a valuable, experienced employee and facing the costs of recruiting and training a replacement.

So it stands to reason there's a good chance you'll be working through perimenopause, menopause and beyond. So where does menopause fit in with your working life? If menopausal symptoms get in the way of you wanting or needing to work, it's time to do something about it.

According to the Faculty of Occupational Medicine, the menopause is rarely discussed in the workplace. And the majority of women are unwilling to disclose menopause-related health problems to their line managers, most of whom are men or younger women.

Line managers have also told us that they have concerns about discussing menopause with women because they feel they do not have enough knowledge or experience of what it's like, telling us that they could get the conversation 'seriously wrong' and cause offence.

Following the publication of the Government Report: Menopause transition: effects on women's economic participation in the UK, published in 2017, this is starting to change. This report pointed out that lack of understanding costs the UK economy millions every year and the need for organisations to take menopause seriously.

More organisations are starting to introduce menopause in the workplace policies and practices, and even for those who don't yet have these in place, menopause is increasingly becoming accepted as an occupational health related issue. So even without a specific menopause policy, you can still ask for help and support from your employer while you come to terms with any symptoms.

As with all things menopause, again it's a case of every woman being different. If you don't notice any symptoms, or they aren't particularly severe, you may just carry on at work as before with no noticeable changes. But for those who are experiencing a host of troublesome symptoms, it can be hard to know where to turn.

Common symptoms women cite include emotional or psychological symptoms such as feeling less than confident about themselves, feeling suddenly emotional, lacking concentration and 'brain fog'.

Then there are the physical symptoms like tiredness and hot flushes, which can be a major source of distress, too. They're not just uncomfortable, they can sometimes be embarrassing, especially when you're meeting with colleagues or clients.

Many have told us that they've not felt able to voice these concerns and often put in place 'coping mechanisms' to hide their symptoms, like writing everything down because they don't trust they'll remember things they'd usually have done with ease before. Others say they simply do not want to admit to any problems or that they're of that age.

Sometimes it's changes at work that can result in a woman not being able to cope any longer – for example, stress can heighten symptoms, or for that matter a change in staff uniform that feels unbearable when a hot flush hits.

Then there's how women are, or believe they're being, treated differently at work. One woman told us that she was fed up about being teased by a colleague whenever she had a hot flush. As she put it 'they wouldn't tease me if I'd been suffering with any other condition, why is it OK to poke fun at me for this?'

So what can you do?

Firstly, nobody wants to be treated differently simply by virtue of being of menopausal age. Nor does anyone want there to be a presumption that their performance will automatically decline at work or they'll be more likely to take time off sick.

But we do need to talk about menopause openly, have help and support when it's needed and continue our careers. It makes good business sense for an employer, too, to retain their valuable investment in their employees, enabling them to perform at their best and reduce the risk of them leaving because they can't cope with work and menopause symptoms.

Remember, maternity policies haven't always been the norm but nowadays no one would question the value of supporting pregnant women or question their ability to do a good job.

It can often be a case of employers making a few small and fairly simple changes to offer support to women and to help them perform to the best of their abilities. These could include incorporating menopause into their policies, talking about it openly, training and education and some small tweaks in their workplace that would make the world of difference.

CONVERSATIONS WITH YOUR EMPLOYER AND LINE MANAGER

It's worth checking if your employer has a menopause policy or other policies in place that could support you. You might find these in your employee handbook or intranet. If so, consider what provision it makes that's relevant to your specific symptoms.

At first glance, these policies may appear to hinder rather than help you – for example, a strict dress code, absence management rules or capability processes. However, some adjustments to these may be reasonable to help manage your symptoms and indeed your employer may have a legal responsibility to do this in order to avoid discrimination linked to age, sex or even disability. There are ways of using these policies to your advantage – for example, by suggesting a referral to Occupational Health to ensure both you and your line manager are getting appropriate support.

Your employer may also have a flexible working policy and in any event, you have a statutory right to formally request flexible working if you've been employed for at least 26 weeks.

How do I have a conversation with my manager about menopause?

If your menopause symptoms are affecting your ability to do your job, how do you broach the subject with your boss?

Let's face it, there may be awkwardness, embarrassment and the fear you won't be taken seriously. It can be hard enough talking to a GP about your symptoms. Many women find it particularly hard to talk to a line manager who may be male, or younger than them, as they feel they won't understand enough about the impact of menopausal symptoms.

So, how do you start a conversation about menopause at work?

First, take a deep breath and remind yourself that your manager is a professional, that there is an increasing awareness about the impact menopause symptoms can have at work, and that you deserve to be listened to.

This simple confident conversation framework can help you get the best possible outcome.

Prepare for your meeting

Keep a diary of your menopause symptoms and how they're affecting you. And also think about the practical, reasonable adjustments that would help you, being flexible and ideally with different options. It may be that these are only for a short period of time while you work with your medical professional to alleviate your symptoms. Include a timeframe, too. This will help you have a much better conversation, resulting in a good outcome for both you and your employer.

Book a time

Booking a meeting means you'll have time and ideally a private office to talk and will be more likely to explain everything in the right way.

Prepare what to say

Mentally rehearse what you're going to say so that when you talk to your boss the words feel and sound natural. You could even do a mini role play with a trusted friend.

Explain your situation clearly

Talk to your boss about your current situation, what's happening and most importantly how it's affecting your work. For example, you're experiencing hot flushes, which are embarrassing you and preventing you from speaking up in meetings. Or night sweats mean you're not sleeping so you're too tired to think clearly and it's taking you longer to make decisions or complete tasks.

Offer a solution

Think about how your circumstances could be improved and offer a reasonable solution. Could you work from home or come into work later on some days if poor sleep is an issue for you? If the temperature in your office is making hot flushes worse, can you have a fan or move to a desk near an air-conditioning unit or a window you can open? Do you have adequate access to drinking water and toilet facilities – if not, how could this be rectified?

Talk these through with your manager and request that some or all of these are put in place as reasonable adjustments, perhaps on a flexible basis so they can be reviewed as appropriate.

Don't expect an answer immediately. Remember, this may have been bothering you for a long time – you've been mentally rehearsing and gathering your courage, but it may be the first time your boss has heard about it. Allow them time to digest the information and seek advice if necessary.

Follow up

At the end of the meeting, put a time in the diary to meet again, whether that's to agree a way forward, to monitor progress or to update.

Above all, remember this is just two professional people having a conversation. It's in both your best interests to find a good solution.

All anyone wants is for you to be fit and well and to do your job to the best of your ability. Menopause can be isolating if you don't talk to someone, but remember all women go through menopause at some point, so you most certainly are not alone.

Why not lead the change, take action and set up an informal or formal support group at work? Arrange to meet regularly with other women in your workplace experiencing similar symptoms and issues, a great opportunity to share your experiences and ease your load.

Sadly, not every employer will be understanding and supportive. If this is the case, consider whether it's appropriate to raise a formal grievance – certainly do this if you feel you are being discriminated against, you are dismissed or your employment contract is otherwise breached (express or implied terms). You may also need to consider bringing a claim in the Employment Tribunal if the treatment towards you breaches employment laws. Please take legal advice at an early stage as strict time limits apply.

If the support you need is a permanent change to your hours, work pattern or place of work, raise a formal flexible working request and ensure this is dealt with in accordance with the ACAS Code (see our **Resources** section).

Menopause doesn't have to be hard work. Talk to your doctor about your options, including HRT, as recommended by the Faculty of Occupational Medicine. And talk to your line manager and colleagues.

WOMEN'S STORIES...

'Menopause wasn't something I ever thought about, until I suddenly noticed my body changing when I was just 39. And the impact it had on my life and career was pretty severe.

I've been a police officer for 15 years, nine of them in the Public Protection Department, which is a very busy place. And to add to my stress, I found I was forgetting what I was supposed to be doing, feeling constantly exhausted and like my energy had been zapped out of me.

I'd gained some weight around my middle, had a sudden onset of headaches, just feeling dreadful all the time for no reason.

My practice nurse suggested I should have a blood test to rule out anything untoward and to confirm that I wasn't going through the menopause. Little did I know that this was actually the beginning of my menopause journey...

The doctor confirmed I had no oestrogen left in my body and this was the cause of why I was feeling so tired. The GP told me I needed to start taking HRT immediately. However, the first lot of HRT made me feel like I had been hit by a bus. The tiredness took over me, the depression started to sneak in... I started to get anxious about going to work.

As months went on, I tried numerous HRTs, patches, tablets. Nothing worked. I would take them for a few weeks and new side effects would appear. The headaches were getting worse. The feelings of not wanting to get out of bed in the mornings were now a permanent fixture. I loved my job but I lost the confidence of who I was. I aspired to be a sergeant in public protection; however, I didn't even know if I wanted to be a police officer any more. I had doubts that I was able to do the job I once loved.

I would spend afternoons staring at my computer screen, feeling exhausted from not sleeping the night before. My concentration levels were at an all-time low.

The hot sweats started and I felt like my whole body was on fire and people could see me getting red. I was a stranger to myself.

I started to research on the intranet about the Force's stance on the menopause. I wanted to find others experiencing what I was going through, so I could talk to them and get a perspective on how they coped with balancing the menopause, shift work, medication and everything else in life.

I could not find any answers but what I did do was begin the conversation... I started to talk about my menopause with anyone who would listen.

It wasn't long before I met with a group of people that were all focused like me and on a mission to change the way the menopause was perceived and handled within the workplace. We needed to make a change in the police force and it needed to happen today. We wanted to raise awareness of the menopause in a positive and productive way.

I became part of a Force working group and I soon found out there was a national menopause working group and it wasn't long before I was sitting around the table representing our Force on the subject.

Hopefully I can encourage others to get talking about the menopause and help them to not feel isolated in the workplace.

I am currently working with others in laying the foundations for our Force guidance on the menopause. We need to educate people and hope that by talking about it we are raising awareness and promoting the menopause in a positive way. Not everybody has a bad time. The menopause affects each woman individually. We need to ensure that there is support for women who do suffer and educate the workplace that line managers may need to look at reasonable adjustments for some females. This is a condition that shall not last forever, I hope.

I refuse to give in to the stigma attached to the menopause, and actively say it is okay to have a bad day and not to feel ashamed or embarrassed. Let's start talking about it!

Our former Chief Constable Sue Fish pledged to support this subject and the work that is going on in the Force around this area... it's time for a change.'

Keeley Mansell

13

....

Menopause: the time of your life

'Embrace the evolution of your life.'
Krys Wojnarowicz

Our mission in producing this guide was to get women talking about menopause. Talking about it with their friends, relatives, work colleagues, doctors and menopause experts. Because life is for living, and as we're living longer and working longer we need to know how to manage this important phase without it becoming overwhelming.

We hope that in these pages you've found some useful information and comfort in reading other women's stories and have learned more about your options, whichever path you think might be best for you.

Perimenopause and menopause needn't take over your life, but by preparing and planning for this transition, you can take control. Nobody should live with distressing or debilitating symptoms and it's important to understand what's happening so you can make informed decisions and seek help from the right places.

Before we started this book, we sent out a survey. In this, we asked women to tell us what their biggest questions about menopause were and what information they'd like to see. And we were heartened that so many of the responses were from women who had already been through menopause and were keen to spread the news that life not only goes on, but can get better. Nobody wants to dismiss the very real and often unpleasant symptoms that menopause brings with it. But by constantly focusing on the negative, we are giving women the unfortunate and misleading impression that they will become old, dried up, forgetful, unattractive and overweight.

It's time to change that.

Let's look at women we at Henpicked admire, leading ladies in the spotlight. Helen Mirren, Judi Dench, Julie Walters, Meryl Streep, Davina McCall, Naomi Campbell, Zoe Ball, Meg Mathews... all vibrant, attractive and successful women. Angelina Jolie went into early menopause after having her ovaries removed and has continued to have a successful career as a prominent actress, campaigner and spokeswoman, along with raising a young family.

So you're menopausal. So what? You've been through puberty and survived. You're about to enter a new phase of your life, and it's up to you how you approach it. And we'll leave you with a quote from our survey that really sums up the whole reason for this book. The reason our initial conversations turned into 'we must do something about this.'

Glossary of Terms

Adrenal glands: help to regulate blood sugar, produce our sex hormones and help to burn fats and proteins.

Adrenaline: a hormone secreted by the adrenal glands that increases breathing rate and activates muscles to take action.

Agonist: a substance that increases the effect of a hormone or chemical messenger.

Antagonist: a substance that reduces the effect of a hormone or chemical messenger.

Bioidentical hormone replacement therapy (BHRT): an unregulated, plant-based hormone replacement therapy, offered on a like-for-like individual basis.

Carbohydrates: one of the three main types of macronutrients; it is changed into glucose (blood sugars) quickly but can increase insulin and, along with cortisol, contributes to fat being laid down around the middle.

Circadian rhythm: internal body clock that regulates our sleep and wake cycle.

Cortisol: a steroid hormone released in response to stress and low blood sugar.

Endocrine system: a collection of glands that produce hormones that regulate metabolism, growth and development, tissue function, sexual function, reproduction, sleep and mood, among other things.

Fragility fracture: a fracture that occurs as a result of normal activities, such as falling from standing height or lower.

FSH (follicle-stimulating hormone): a hormone that makes the egg grow in the follicle in the ovary.

Good fats: foods that are high in monounsaturated fat, such as olive oil, avocado and nuts.

HIIT: high intensity interval training for a short period of time with less intense recovery periods.

Hormone: a chemical substance produced by our bodies that controls and regulates the activity of certain cells or organs. Hormones are essential throughout our lives and for every activity of life, including growth, reproduction and mood control.

Menopause: 12 months after your last period.

Muscle density: this refers to the concentration of muscle fibres within a muscle. An increased density usually correlates to increased strength.

Muscle mass: the amount of skeletal muscle tissue found in the body, also referred to as muscle strength. Other types of muscle include 'smooth' muscle, which forms your gut walls and sphincters throughout the body and can also deteriorate with age and hormonal change.

Nutrient-dense foods: foods rich in a variety of nutrients, including vitamins and minerals.

Oestradiol/estradiol: the strongest and most active form of oestrogen.

Oestriol/estriol: the weakest form of oestrogen, produced in the placenta during pregnancy.

Oestrogen/estrogen: the primary female hormone responsible for maintaining your reproductive system, as well as other organs.

Oestrone/estrone: another form of oestrogen, produced at the time of the menopause, which our bodies convert to oestradiol.

Perimenopause: the time leading up to menopause.

Phytoestrogens: plant-based foods that can exert a naturally oestrogenic effect upon your body.

Premature ovarian insufficiency (POI): menopause that occurs before the age of 40, which can happen as a result of medical or surgical intervention or occur naturally.

Processed foods: commercially produced foods such as pizza, cupcakes and ready meals that often contain trans fats.

Progesterone: a hormone that plays a major part in your reproductive health.

Protein: by far the most thermogenic of the three macronutrients (protein, carbohydrates and fat), found in foods such as chicken, turkey, fish, dairy, eggs, lentils, nuts.

Self-hypnosis: a way to manage your thoughts, and build yourself up from the inside.

Serotonin: a chemical in the body that plays a role in improving mood.

SSRI (Selective Seratonin Reuptake Inhibitor): a form of antidepressant.

Stress management: a set of tools or strategies to reduce, prevent or cope with stress.

Testosterone: a male hormone also important for women, which is mostly converted into oestrogen by female enzymes.

Thermogenic: the process by which your body burns calories from the food you have just eaten, turning them into heat/energy.

Acknowledgements

We'd like to thank the experts for their hard work and practical advice.

Dr Louise Newson BSc (Hons), MBChB (Hons), MRCP, FRCGP

Dr Louise Newson trained in Manchester, Southampton and New Zealand and is a GP in Solihull, West Midlands. She runs a private menopause clinic at Spire Parkway Hospital, Solihull.

Louise feels passionately about trying to improve awareness of safe prescribing of HRT to healthcare professionals and women, and has written many articles and editorials and given local and national presentations on this subject. She strongly feels that women should be offered the correct information about treatment options so they can make an informed choice regarding management of their menopause.

She is the West Midlands lead for the Primary Care Women's Health Forum. She is a member of the International Menopause Society and the British Menopause Society. Louise works regularly with West Midlands Police and West Midlands Fire Service to provide advice and support regarding menopause in the workplace.

Kathryn Peden BSc (Hons), HCPC, MCSP, MPOGP

Kathryn found her passion for physiotherapy after working in corporate training, photography, and social care and health for a number of years. Having worked with older people, she developed a skill not just for rehabilitating people with a wide range of injuries, but for encouraging knowledge and interest in the human body and promoting wellness for life.

This has come to the fore even further with her specialism, women's health physiotherapy. Determined to tackle society's mantra to women's troubles – 'That's just being a mum' – she helps women both pre- and postnatal understand their own bodies, why they are in pain or having issues with their bladder, tummy or back, and guiding them down the road to full postnatal recovery, putting the woman first and securing knowledge for future pregnancies. Kathryn also works with women who don't have children but still encounter specifically female issues, perhaps with painful sex, post-surgery scars or rehabilitation, or urinary leakage on activity.

Kathryn does public speaking on a range of physical health topics such as posture, well-being and postnatal education, and is a contributor to Henpicked.net, as well as regularly writing her own blogs.

Katherine Bellchambers BSc, MNIMH

Katherine is a medical herbalist. She trained first at the College of Phytotherapy and graduated with BSc Honours in Herbal Medicine from the University of East London. She has many years of experience and specialises in the treatment of hormonal imbalance that assails women throughout their lives. From puberty to menopause and beyond, these pesky substances influence our lives. Katherine uses herbs and offers dietary and lifestyle advice to help women take control of their health to feel their best and live life to the full. As well as practising herbal medicine directly with patients, she grows herbs, makes medicine and writes extensively on herbal medicine and women's health. She also acts as an advisor for a number of publications and serves as a director of the National Institute of Medical Herbalists.

Pamela Windle BSc (Hons), Dip Hyp, GHR Reg, GQHP

Pamela is an experienced women's health therapist who is passionate about transforming women's lives as they unfold their unique hormonal journey.

She strongly believes that the perimenopause, menopause and beyond doesn't need to be as debilitating as we are led to believe and that we can age gracefully, remaining strong, healthy and happy in body and mind.

She holds numerous qualifications, including an advanced certificate in 3rd Age Practitioner, Women's Health Coach Certification, a BSc Psychology with Sports Science and a combined Hypnotherapy and Psychotherapy diploma, and is a qualified Certified Hypnotic Birthing Practitioner (CHBP). She is a qualified personal trainer and has worked since 2000 in the field. She effortlessly brings these disciplines together to create a holistic (and fun) path towards whole body healing.

Diane Danzebrink

Diane is passionate about empowering women to take control of their health and well-being. As a result of her own menopause experience, which had a profound effect on her quality of life for a period of time, she created a national support service for women and those who love them to access advice, guidance, evidence-based information and emotional support. She has completed the menopause foundations course for nurses and is the media lay spokesperson for the Royal College of Obstetricians and Gynaecologists and a member of the Women's Voices involvement panel. Diane is also a member of and ambassador for the British Menopause Society. She is a passionate campaigner and advocate for improved care of and support for women experiencing menopause both in and out of the workplace. Diane works as a women's health and well-being coach, trauma therapist and mind management trainer. Along with her private clients, she leads menopause workshops and educational training for therapists and organisations.

Clare Shepherd DipNHF, FNTP

A full hysterectomy in her 30s led nutritional therapist and health coach Clare on an amazing adventure, exploring the many opportunities available to manage her enforced menopause and create long-term health. Clare prefers the natural approach, and qualifying in nutritional therapy gave her the confidence to come off HRT, take back control of her life and health, and look forward to living the best third of her life free of prescription drugs. Understanding the importance of creating harmony of health of both body and mind through menopause and beyond, she's now on a mission to inspire, educate and empower other women, too.

Julie Dennis

Julie is a nutrition adviser and qualified level 4 personal trainer with a City and Guilds Introduction to Trainer Skills qualification.

She specialises in practical and natural solutions for controlling menopause symptoms and helps busy professional women break through the brain fog of menopause.

She is an experienced speaker and has been quoted in the national press to raise awareness around menopause.

The combination of her personal experience and business background means she is well placed to understand the needs of both private individuals and business.

Lester Aldridge LLP

Lester Aldridge is a full-service law firm for businesses and individuals. Their specialist Employment Law team have a strong understanding of how stressful disagreements or disputes in the workplace can be, and how to resolve them. The team can explain what treatment you can and should expect in the workplace, and can offer you practical legal advice to resolve a wide range of employment and HR issues.

Relate

Relate is the UK's largest provider of relationship support, and every year nationally helps over a million people of all ages, backgrounds and sexual orientations to strengthen their relationships. Relationships with family, partners, friends and colleagues play a big part in how happy we are.

Alison Towner has been working at Relate for 14 years and is a Relationship Counsellor, Psychosexual Therapist and Supervisor. She also works in the NHS and has been involved with training psychosexual therapists. Jo Glazebrook, Centre Manager for Relate Nottinghamshire, is passionate about leading an organisation that promotes the importance of strengthening relationships.

Dr Karen Morton

Dr Karen Morton is a consultant gynaecologist and obstetrician working at the Royal Surrey County Hospital in Guildford. Karen worked in general medicine and intensive neonatal care before undertaking specialist training in Oxford, Cambridge, Queen Charlotte's Hospital and St Thomas', London.

Realising that medicine had been slow to embrace communication technology, she set up a medical helpline service offering immediate access to expert medical advice. Through this, she hopes to address a gender health inequality – as women need, for gynaecological reasons (menopause, contraception, period problems, fertility and pregnancy), to seek medical advice 42 per cent more than men.

Special thanks for their time and expertise go to:

Dr Marilyn Glenville PhD

Dr Marilyn Glenville is the UK's leading nutritionist specialising in women's health. She is the former President of the Food and Health Forum at the Royal Society of Medicine, a registered nutritionist, psychologist, author and popular broadcaster who obtained her doctorate from Cambridge University. Dr Glenville is a popular international speaker and the author of 14 internationally bestselling books, including *Natural Solutions to Menopause*.

The Glenville Nutrition Clinics are in Harley Street, London and Tunbridge Wells, Kent; and also have practices in Dublin, Cork, Galway and Kilkenny in Ireland.

Dr Heather Currie MB BS, FRCOG, DRCOG, MRCGP

Dr Currie is an Associate Specialist Gynaecologist and Obstetrician, at Dumfries and Galloway Royal Infirmary, Dumfries. She is Managing Director of Menopause Matters Limited and former Chair of British Menopause Society.

Dr Sarah Gray

Dr Sarah Gray is a GP from Cornwall, where she provides clinical leadership for contraception and sexual health. She has run an NHS menopause referral service drawing patients from a wide geographical area.

She teaches nationally and has a long list of publications that focus on applying the latest research in women's health to primary care. She was a member of the groups who developed NICE guidance and quality standards for heavy menstrual bleeding.

Her wider role includes medical politics, a regular phone-in on BBC local radio and as a team leader for the Fitness to Practise directorate of the General Medical Council. She can see women both privately and in Truro and Plymouth.

Dr Marian Everett MB, ChB, FFSRH

Dr Everett retired earlier this year from her position as a consultant in sexual and reproductive health. She has been involved with women's health for more than 30 years, 20 years in Leeds and the last 13 years in Hull and East Yorkshire, where she was the consultant menopause lead.

She is a member of the Medical Advisory Council of the British Menopause Society and the Council of the Faculty of Sexual and Reproductive Health. She is the Faculty Guardian of the

Special Skills Module in Menopause, a joint training programme developed by the BMS and Faculty for doctors and nurses. She has been involved in teaching and education, particularly in menopause and contraception, for many years and is passionate about providing up-to-date evidence-based information so other health professionals can advise women and their families and allow them to make informed choices about their management options.

Dr Marion Gluck

Dr Marion Gluck trained as a medical doctor in Hamburg more than 30 years ago and has worked all over the world as a women's health specialist. She is passionate about the potential of bioidentical hormones to change the lives of women and men for the better. It is her life's work to educate people about hormonal imbalance.

Julia Church

Julia is a qualified and experienced massage therapist, passionate about nurturing the whole being through massage and common-sense nutritional advice. She serves women from pre-pregnancy to menopause and beyond. She believes in eating real food as much as possible to aid in healing and recovery and to cleanse our bodies, minds and souls.

The Henpicked Team
Deborah Garlick, founder of Henpicked.net and Menopause In The Workplace

Deborah is passionate about helping thousands and thousands of women live better lives by raising awareness and understanding around the menopause, changing perceptions and getting everyone talking about it.

She is the founder of Henpicked.net which, since its launch, has grown to be one of the UK's largest, fastest-growing communities for women over 40, providing a platform for women to help one another by sharing their wisdom, stories, tips and support.

Since 2016 she has been working with employers to help them understand how menopause affects women at work, raising awareness and helping them educate their colleagues and line managers. Menopause In The Workplace was launched in 2017.

Kay Garrett, editor of Henpicked.net

Kay is a writer and editor with over 20 years' experience. As Henpicked's editor, she enjoys reading stories from women across the globe, from all walks of life, all experiencing similar life events.

She believes that women can learn so much from each other about how to manage their menopause by talking about and sharing their experiences.

Resources

Henpicked.net

One of the UK's largest, fastest-growing communities for women over 40. Join us for more articles and conversations about menopause and life at:

www.henpicked.net/menopause

www.facebook.com/henpickedcommunity

www.twitter.com/henpickednet

www.menopauseintheworkplace.co.uk

CONTRIBUTORS AND EXPERTS' WEBSITES

Dr Louise Newson

GP and menopause expert: www.menopausedoctor.co.uk

Kathryn Peden

Physiotherapist: www.arcadia-therapy.com

Katherine Bellchambers

Medical herbalist: www.nottingham-herbalist.co.uk

Pamela Windle

Women's health therapist: www.smarterchange.co.uk

Dr Marilyn Glenville

The UK's leading nutritionist specialising in women's health: www.marilynglenville.com and www.naturalhealthpractice.com

Clare Shepherd

Nutritional therapist and menopause coach: www. yournewlifeplan.com

Julie Dennis

Menopause coach, nutritional adviser and PT instructor: www. juliedennis.net

Dr Karen Morton

Consultant gynaecologist, obstetrician, Founder and Medical Director at Dr Morton's - the medical helpline: www.drmortons. co.uk

Dr Sarah Gray

GP specialist in women's health: www.drsarahgray.co.uk

Dr Marion Gluck

Women's health and BHRT specialist: www.mariongluckclinic. com

Jo Divine

Sam Evans is a writer and commentator on all things sexual – especially for women over 40, including luxury sex toys and vibrators: www.jodivine.com.

WEBSITES FOR MENOPAUSE INFORMATION

The National Institute for Health and Care Excellence (NICE)
Provides national guidance and advice to improve health and social care:
www.nice.org.uk/guidance/ng23/ifp/chapter/About-this-information

The Daisy Network
Provides information and support to women with Premature Ovarian Insufficiency (POI), also known as Premature Menopause:
www.daisynetwork.org.uk

International Menopause Society
Promotes knowledge, study and research on all aspects of ageing in women: www.imsociety.org

British Menopause Society
Provides education, information and guidance to healthcare professionals specialising in all aspects of post-reproductive health: www.thebms.org.uk

Women's Health Concern
The patient arm of the British Menopause Society (BMS), providing an independent service to advise, reassure and educate women of all ages about their health, wellbeing and lifestyle concerns: www.womens-health-concern.org

Menopause Matters
Provides information for healthcare professionals and patients: www.menopausematters.co.uk

How to find if there's a menopause clinic in your area: www.menopausematters.co.uk/clinicfinder.php

National Institute of Medical Herbalists

How to find a herbalist in your area: www.nimh.org.uk/find-a-herbalist/

Menopause in the Workplace
Advice and services for employers and colleagues

Specialist advice and information on policies, raising awareness and training, providing expert menopause speakers: www.menopauseintheworkplace.co.uk

Government Equalities Office Report, Menopause transition: effects on women's economic participation

Provides information following in-depth research on the reasons why employers need to take menopause seriously: https://www.gov.uk/government/publications/menopause-transition-effects-on-womens-economic-participation

Faculty of Occupational Medicine guidelines (FOM)

Provides useful information on what employers can do: www.fom.ac.uk/health-at-work-2/information-for-employers/dealing-with-health-problems-in-the-workplace/advice-on-the-menopause

Lester Aldridge LLP

Full-service law firm for businesses and individuals: www.lesteraldridge.com

ACAS

Provides information, advice, training, conciliation and other services for employers and employees: www.acas.org.uk

RELATIONSHIPS, MINDFULNESS AND SOCIAL EVENTS

Relate

The UK's largest provider of relationship support: www.relate.org.uk

Menopause Café

A Menopause Café is a group-directed discussion of menopause, with no agenda, objectives or themes. Rolling out across the country, you can attend or organise one: www.menopausecafe.net

British Association for Behavioural & Cognitive Psychotherapies (BABCP)

Find out how to access behavioural and cognitive psychotherapy: www.babcp.com

British Psychological Society (BPS)

Learn about psychology, the work that psychologists do, and how to find a psychologist if you need support: www.bps.org.uk

Mindfulness Association

Provides training and resources in mindfulness: www.mindfulnessassociation.net

Index

acne   15
alcohol   13, 30, 37, 52, 128, 145
Alzheimer's disease   115
anger   16, 42
antidepressants   37, 47
anxiety   16, 132, 145
autoimmune disease   143

belly breathing   37, 43–4, 86
belly fat   47–50
BHRT (bioidentical hormone
    replacement therapy)
    123–5
bilateral oophorectomy
    (BSO)   149
black cohosh (*Actaea racemosa*)
    132–3
bleeding, vaginal   61, 82, 112
blessed thistle (*Cnicus benedictus*)
    132
blood clots   118, 121
blood pressure   147
blood sugar levels   30, 38
bones   23, 65–6, 67–8
  bone density   27, 69, 144
bowel cancer   115
boxing   73
breast cancer   115–17, 146
breast pain   14

breathing techniques   37, 42,
    43–5, 85–6
BSO (bilateral oophorectomy)
    149

caffeine   52, 69, 87
calcium   69, 72
cancer   111–12, 115–17, 143, 146
carbohydrates: reduction of
    intake   126–7
cardiovascular disease   114–15,
    116, 118, 121, 146, 147, 150
cardiovascular exercise   38, 72
CBT (cognitive behavioural
    therapy)   46
chemotherapy   11, 143
cholesterol   23, 28, 114–15, 147
communication   45, 157–66
  with partners   158–63, 164
complementary therapies   129–31
concentration: low levels of   16
contraception   17, 18, 31,
    59–60, 146
cortisol (stress hormone)   28, 37,
    38, 48, 86, 126
cystitis   16

Daisy Network   148
dancing   73

deep vein thrombosis
    (DVT)   118
dementia   115
depression   16, 132, 145
DEXA scan (bone density
    test)   144
diet   28–9, 30, 38, 49, 50, 96,
    125–8, 145
dietary fat   28, 128
dizziness   13
doctors: appointments
    with   173–7
DVT (deep vein thrombosis)   118

early menopause   11, 140–1,
    150: *see also* premature ovarian
    insufficiency (POI); surgical
    menopause
emotional symptoms   16, 39–47
    medical approaches to   46–7
    natural approaches to   41–6
    retreat from everyday life   40–1
    see also mood swings
emotions: as inner guidance
    system   43
episiotomies   98–9
ethnicity   11
exercise   29, 37–8, 49, 70, 71–3,
    128–9, 145

facial hair growth   15
falls   70–1
flexible working   187
fragility fractures   68

FSH (follicle stimulating
    hormone)   17, 23

hair: changes in   15
heart attacks   114, 121, 146,
    147, 150
heart palpitations   13
heavy periods   61–3
herbal therapies   129–31
high blood pressure   147
HIIT (high intensity interval
    training)   38, 128–9
hops (*Humulus lupus*)   133
hormone replacement therapy,
    see HRT
hormones   17, 21–30, 65–6,
    126, 128
    balancing   27–30
    bioidentical hormones
        (BHRT)   123–5
    body-identical hormones   125
    fluctuating levels, results of   12,
        14, 15, 21–2, 24, 48
    medical approaches to
        balancing   30–1
    natural approaches to
        balancing   27–30
    post-hysterectomy   150–1
    and sleep problems   51, 52
    stress hormones   28, 37, 38,
        48, 86, 126
    see also HRT (hormone replace-
        ment therapy); oestrogens;
        progestogens; testosterone

hot flushes   13, 18, 36–8, 131
HRT (hormone replacement
    therapy)   30–1, 37, 46–7,
    50, 51, 62, 109–22
    benefits of   113–14
    and cancer   111–12, 115–17,
    146
    and cardiovascular
        disease   114–17, 121
    combined (oestrogen and
        progestogen)   117
    facts about   120–2
    and lessening sex drive
        (libido)   95
    and Mirena coil   62
    NICE guidelines   110, 115,
    118
    oestrogen-only   117
    and POI   145–6
    post-hysterectomy   150–1
    and pregnancy   60
    risks of   115–18, 121, 146
    side effects   118–19
    and stress incontinence   85
    types of   111–13
    and vaginal dryness   82, 114
human growth hormone   128
hydration   127
hysterectomy   11, 143, 149

immune system   143
incontinence   28, 79, 83–90
    medical approaches to   84–5
    natural approaches to   85–7

stress incontinence   83–5, 87,
    88–9
urge incontinence   84, 85,
    87, 89
itching   15, 80

joint pain   16
journal keeping   45–6

Kegel exercises   85–7, 88, 90, 96,
    101–2

libido (sex drive)   13, 94–6,
    99–100, 163–4
life changes   166
ligaments   68–9
light
    blue light from devices   51
    natural light   29
light-headedness   13
lubricants   82–3

Marigold (*Calendula
    officinalis*)   133
masturbation   100–1
medical approaches to
    emotional symptoms   46–7
    excess belly fat   50
    heavy periods   62–3
    hormonal changes   30–1
    hot flushes   37
    incontinence   84–5
    lessening sex drive
        (libido)   95

vaginal dryness 81–2
see also HRT (hormone
   replacement therapy)
meditation 37, 42, 49
memory problems 14
menopause
   age at which it occurs 9, 10–12
   diagnosis of 17–18
   men's perceptions 167–8
Menopause Cafes 45
menopause clinics 177, 209
menopause management
   medical approaches to 109–25
   natural approaches to 125–6
micronised progesterone 113, 116
migraines 15, 121
milk thistle (*Silybum*
   marianum) 132
mindfulness meditation 42
Mirena coils 31, 62–3, 112
missed periods 18
mood swings 14, 39, 46–7,
   161
muscle pain 16

natural approaches to:
   emotional symptoms 41–6
   excess belly fat 49–50
   hormonal changes 27–30
   hot flushes 37–8
   incontinence 85–7
   lessening sex drive (libido) 95–6
   menopause management 125–6
   vaginal dryness 82–3

NICE (National Institute of
   Health and Care Excellence)
   guidelines 110–11, 115,
   118, 123, 129, 150, 173–4
night sweats 13, 18, 131
NLP (Neuro-Linguistic
   Programming) 42

obesity: risks of 118
oestrogens 11, 22–4, 26, 30,
   81, 149
   changes caused by decrease
      in 14, 15, 16, 79–80
   oestradiol 24, 112, 131, 151
   oestriol 24
   oestrone 24
   phytoestrogens 28–9, 127,
      131
   and urge incontinence 85
   and weight gain 48
   see also HRT (hormone
      replacement therapy)
oophorectomy 143, 149
osteoporosis 27, 29, 67–8, 115,
   145, 146–7, 150
ovarian surgery 11: *see also*
   POI (premature ovarian
   insufficiency)

painful intercourse (dyspareunia)
   14, 80, 164
panic attacks 16
PE (pulmonary embolism) 118
pelvic floor dysfunction 86, 87

pelvic floor exercises   85–7, 88, 90, 96, 101–2
pelvic floor muscles   84, 96–9
peony root (*Paeonia lactiflora*)   132
perimenopause   8–9
  contraception in   59–60
  hormonal fluctuations   24
  pregnancy in   59–60
  symptoms   12–16
periods   57–63
  bleeding after cessation of   61
  changes in   12, 57–9
  heavy periods   61–3
  missed periods   18
phytoestrogens   28–9, 127, 131
PMS (premenstrual syndrome)   12
POI (premature ovarian insufficiency)   140, 142–8
positive thoughts   44
positive visualisation   37, 42
postmenopause   18
posture   68–9
pregnancy   59–60, 131, 142
premature ovarian insufficiency (POI)   140, 142–8
premenstrual syndrome (PMS)   12
progestogens   111–12, 113
  micronised progesterone   113, 116
  progesterone   24, 25–6, 149
pulmonary embolism (PE)   118

radiotherapy   11, 143
red clover (*Trifolium praetens*)   131

red raspberry leaf (*Rubus idaeus*)   133
reflection   43–6
relaxation techniques   37
resistance training   72

sage (*Salvia officinalis*)   131
St John's wort (*Hypericum perforatum*)   132
same-sex partners   163
self-care   40–1, 43–6
self-consciousness   161–2
self-hypnosis   37
self-image: importance of   66
sex drive (libido)   13, 94–6, 99–100, 163–4
sexual intercourse   82, 84, 96, 97
  painful intercourse (dyspareunia)   14, 80, 164
sexual problems   165
sexually transmitted diseases: protection from   59–60, 62
skin: changes in   15
sleep problems   13–14, 51–2
smoking   11, 52, 70, 145
social media: and sleep problems   51
spinal ligaments   68
spotting   58, 112
stress   18, 28, 37, 49, 126
stress incontinence   83–5, 87, 88–9
strokes   118, 121, 147
sugar: reduction of intake   126–7

supplements   128, 129, 145
support groups   45, 187
surgical menopause   148–52
sweating   13
swimming   73

TAH (total hysterectomy)   149
testosterone   26–7, 95, 119, 132,
    149, 151–2
thrush   15, 80, 82
tiredness   51–2
total hysterectomy (TAH)   149
tribulus (*Tribulus terrestris*)   132

urge incontinence   84, 85, 87, 89
urinary symptoms   16
urination: frequency of   89
UTIs (urinary tract infections)
    16, 79–80, 82, 114

vagina: look and feel of   89–90,
    100–2
vaginal bleeding   61, 82, 112

vaginal dryness   14–15, 18,
    78–83, 95, 114
    medical approaches to   81–2
    natural approaches to   82–3
vaginal itching   15, 80
vaginal ring pessaries   84
vaginal soreness   15
vaginismus   164
venous thromboembolism   118
vitamin D   29, 145

weight gain   14, 18, 47–50
weight loss   18
working life   180–7
    employment law breaches   187
    flexible working   187
    menopause policies   180,
        182–4
    support groups   187
    talking to line managers
        184–7

yoga   37, 44–5, 49, 73